DERMATOLOGY - LABORATORY AND CLINICAL RESEARCH

PSORIASIS: CAUSES, TREATMENTS AND PATHOLOGICAL MODELS

DERMATOLOGY - LABORATORY AND CLINICAL RESEARCH

Additional books in this series can be found on Nova's website under the Series tab.

Additional E-books in this series can be found on Nova's website under the E-book tab.

DERMATOLOGY - LABORATORY AND CLINICAL RESEARCH

PSORIASIS: CAUSES, TREATMENTS AND PATHOLOGICAL MODELS

JESSICA JEAN
MARTHA ESTRELLA GARCIA-PÉREZ
SIMON GUÉRARD
AND
ROXANE POULIOT

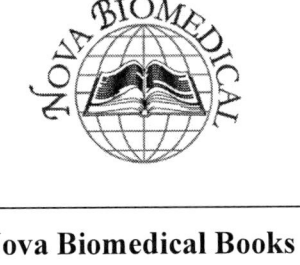

Nova Biomedical Books
New York

Copyright © 2011 by Nova Science Publishers, Inc.

All rights reserved. No part of this book may be reproduced, stored in a retrieval system or transmitted in any form or by any means: electronic, electrostatic, magnetic, tape, mechanical photocopying, recording or otherwise without the written permission of the Publisher.

For permission to use material from this book please contact us:
Telephone 631-231-7269; Fax 631-231-8175
Web Site: http://www.novapublishers.com

NOTICE TO THE READER

The Publisher has taken reasonable care in the preparation of this book, but makes no expressed or implied warranty of any kind and assumes no responsibility for any errors or omissions. No liability is assumed for incidental or consequential damages in connection with or arising out of information contained in this book. The Publisher shall not be liable for any special, consequential, or exemplary damages resulting, in whole or in part, from the readers' use of, or reliance upon, this material. Any parts of this book based on government reports are so indicated and copyright is claimed for those parts to the extent applicable to compilations of such works.

Independent verification should be sought for any data, advice or recommendations contained in this book. In addition, no responsibility is assumed by the publisher for any injury and/or damage to persons or property arising from any methods, products, instructions, ideas or otherwise contained in this publication.

This publication is designed to provide accurate and authoritative information with regard to the subject matter covered herein. It is sold with the clear understanding that the Publisher is not engaged in rendering legal or any other professional services. If legal or any other expert assistance is required, the services of a competent person should be sought. FROM A DECLARATION OF PARTICIPANTS JOINTLY ADOPTED BY A COMMITTEE OF THE AMERICAN BAR ASSOCIATION AND A COMMITTEE OF PUBLISHERS.

Additional color graphics may be available in the e-book version of this book.

LIBRARY OF CONGRESS CATALOGUING-IN-PUBLICATION DATA

Psoriasis : causes, treatments, and pathological models / Jessica Jean ... [et al.].
    p. ; cm.
  Includes bibliographical references and index.
  ISBN 978-1-61209-691-9 (softcover : alk. paper)
  1. Psoriasis. I. Jean, Jessica.
  [DNLM: 1. Psoriasis. WR 205]   RL321.P6756 2011   616.5'26--dc22

Published by Nova Science Publishers, Inc. † New York

Contents

Preface		vii
List of Abbreviations		ix
Chapter I	Psoriasis	1
Chapter II	Causes of Psoriasis	7
Chapter III	Treatments of Psoriasis	23
Chapter IV	Pathological Models of Psoriasis	33
Chapter V	Advances of Concepts on the Pathogenesis of Psoriasis	39
Chapter VI	Conclusion	43
Acknowledgements		45
References		47
Index		67

Preface

Psoriasis is a common, inflammatory, multi-systemic skin disease characterized by hyper-proliferation and abnormal differentiation of epidermis. It affects approximately 2% of the world's population, both men and women, aged between 15 and 30 years. Psoriasis is typically recognized with sharply demarcated red, scaly dermatological plaques affecting most body surfaces but especially knees, elbows and scalp. Generally, psoriasis is not a fatal disease, but the presence of physical and psychological pains can severely affect patients' quality of life.

There is a wide variety of therapeutic options to treat psoriasis, including topical, phototherapy, systemic and biological therapies.

These treatments can control or prevent symptoms; however, there is still no cure available. During the past decade, many pathological models have been developed to better understand psoriasis. Among them, *in vitro* models offer an interesting alternative to animal ones. Their development represents a key component in the fight against psoriasis.

This complete review of psoriasis presents the characteristics of this pathology, the suggested causes, the treatments (side effects and mechanisms of action) and the current state of research on pathological models to better understand mechanisms of psoriasis.

List of Abbreviations

CAT	catalase
CD	cluster of differentiation
GPx	glutathione peroxidase
GM-CSF	granulocyte macrophage colony-stimulating factor
HLA-DR	human leukocyte antigen class II
ICAM	intercellular adhesion molecule
IFN	interferon
Ig	immunoglobulin
IL	interleukin
K	keratin
LFA	lymphocyte function-associated antigen
MHC	major histocompatibility complex
NK	natural killer cells
NO	nitric oxide
PASI	psoriasis area and severity index
RAR	retinoic acid receptor
ROS	reactive oxygen species
SC	*stratum corneum*
SCID	severe combined immunodeficient mice
SOD	superoxide dismutase
Th	T helper cells
TNF	tumor necrosis factor
VEGF	vascular endothelial growth factor

Chapter I

Psoriasis

History

Psoriasis is probably one of the longest known human illnesses but, even today, this pathology is not well understood. Psoriasis was described throughout history as a kind of leprosy. In the late 18th century, it became known as Willan's lepra when English dermatologists Robert Willan and Thomas Bateman differentiated it from other skin diseases [1]. However, Willan also wrote about another skin condition, which he called psoriasis. In 1841, this skin disorder was finally named "psoriasis" by the dermatologist Ferdinand von Hebra. The name was derived from the Greek word *psora*, which means "to itch" [2].

Prevalence

The prevalence of psoriasis is estimated to be around 2% [3]. It varies depending on the geographic region and the population groups studied. Thus, in a study of twin pairs in Australia, it was demonstrated that psoriasis occurred more frequently in southern states than in the warmer northern states [4]. Similarly, a study in Norway noted that higher prevalence rates of psoriasis are observed in the northern and cooler parts of the country and lower rates in the southern regions [5]. Additionally, several studies have indicated that ethnic factors, such as genetic and behavioral factors, may influence the prevalence of psoriasis [6]. For instance, the frequency ranges are 0% in the Samoan population to nearly 12.0% in Arctic Kazach'ye [7]. In the United States, the prevalence of psoriasis in white American population is estimated to 2.5%, whereas in African Americans it is only 1.3% [8]. Data for prevalence in Europe including the United Kingdom, Norway and Croatia shows small variations. Thus, it ranges from 1.6% (United Kingdom), 1.4% (Norway) and 1.6% (Croatia) [3]. In East Africa, the prevalence of psoriasis is 0.7%, while in the Henan district of China it is only 0.4% [7].

Most studies also suggest that psoriasis is slightly more prevalent among men than women [9]. Effectively, a systematic survey conducted in Denmark showed that the prevalence of psoriasis for men was 4.2%, while the prevalence for women was 3.3% [10]. However, in patients under 20 years old, the prevalence of psoriasis was greater in women than in men, suggesting an earlier onset age of psoriasis in women [11-12]. Moreover, prevalence data of psoriasis reveals that the frequency of psoriasis decreases in older individuals [11, 13]. This decrease has not been elucidated. However, Neimann et al. have proposed three possible explanations: first, remission could be observed in older individuals; second, they do not come to medical attention and, consequently, are not captured by medical approaches measuring prevalence and finally, a higher mortality rate from associated comorbidities and risky behaviors could explain the decrease [6].

Types of Psoriasis

Distinct types of psoriasis exist, and they are regrouped within the general term "psoriasis". The classification proposed is based solely on the phenotype and is intended to be used both in clinic and research [14-16]. Although phenotype-based, those different types of psoriasis can also differ in their pathogenesis and, therefore, treatment options.

Plaque Psoriasis

Plaque psoriasis is by far the most common type (about 90%) [17]. In fact, plaque psoriasis is sometimes referred as simply "psoriasis". Phenotypically, it is characterized by red, scaly plaques with a diameter of at least 0.5 cm. Also, the distinction between plaques and normal skin is usually very clear. These plaques are sometimes more active at the edge, which can lead to an annular shape with normal skin in the middle and affected skin on the border. Plaques are often symmetrically distributed over the body. This distribution is variable between patients, but some areas are more likely to be affected (e.g., elbows, knees and scalp) than some others (e.g., face). In fact, a sub-classification following the region affected exists (flexural psoriasis, nail psoriasis, scalp psoriasis, palmoplantar psoriasis and sebopsoriasis). This sub-classification is clinically very important to guide clinicians in the treatment.

Guttate Psoriasis

Guttate psoriasis is an acute form of psoriasis in which small papules erupt on the trunk, the limbs or the face. It often appears following a streptococcal infection.

Pustular Psoriasis

Pustular psoriasis, as its name implies, is the apparition of small pustules appearing either at the edge or in the middle of an existing inflammatory plaque.

Erythrodermic Psoriasis

Erythrodermic psoriasis is characterized by the acute apparition of a diffusely red, inflammatory patch covering almost the entire body surface (90% or more). In comparison to plaque psoriasis flares, where large and very thick plaques appear, patients suffering from erythrodermic psoriasis will have fewer plaques and those will not be as thick.

Severity of Psoriasis

Severity of psoriasis is assessed by how much body surface area the disease covers and is frequently classified as mild, moderate and severe. The gold standard for the assessment of extensive psoriasis is the Psoriasis Area and Severity Index (PASI), which was developed in 1978, by Fredricksson and Pettersson for use in a clinical trial [18]. The PASI is a measure of average redness, thickness and scaliness of the lesions (graded on a 0 to 4 scale) and considers the area of involvement, thereby resulting in a single score for psoriasis severity [19]. Recently, the pharmaceutical companies and the US Food and Drug Administration have considered a reduction from baseline PASI score of ≥ 75% (PASI 75), as a primary endpoint in clinical trials in order to assess the effectiveness of anti-psoriatic treatments [20-21]. In fact, patients reaching PASI 75 show important improvements in psoriasis severity and in their quality of life [22]. Even if PASI is the most commonly used measure of psoriasis severity in clinical trials, it does have a number of limitations [19]. For instance, PASI is rarely used by dermatologists in clinical practice [22]. Moreover, PASI has a poor sensitivity to change for relatively small areas of involvement. Thus, in studies involving treatment for small plaques, target lesion assessments are generally preferred [19].

Histological Features

The histology of psoriatic skin reveals numerous hallmarks of the pathology including (1) hyperplasia of the epidermis, (2) accumulation of inflammatory cells in the skin and (3) increased angiogenesis [17].

First, a pronounced thickening of the epidermis is observed in psoriatic skin, illustrating the hyperproliferation of keratinocytes [23]. Also, there is an elongation of the epidermal *rete* at the dermo-epidermal junction. On the other hand, the altered maturation of keratinocytes is reflected by the shivering or the absence of the granular layer, in which keratinocytes would normally enter terminal differentiation. This incomplete terminal differentiation leads to the presence of nucleated cells in the SC, a specific hallmark of psoriasis [24] (Figure 1). Those alterations in the epidermis result in an immature skin, which has an increased permeability.

Second, an important accumulation of inflammatory cells in both the dermis and the epidermis demonstrates the inflammatory nature of psoriasis itself. A wide variety of inflammatory cells can be found, including both polymorphonuclear (neutrophils) and mononuclear leukocytes (T lymphocytes, monocytes and dendritic cells) [23, 25]. Accumulation of neutrophils in the SC is known as Munro's microabscesses and is specific to psoriasis [26]. These inflammatory cells have an increased adherence in psoriatic skin and are believed to have a crucial part in the disease's pathogenesis [25].

Finally, blood vessels in psoriatic plaques are abnormal. Their size and their number are significantly increased [27-28]. This dilatation of blood vessels would be responsible for the redness of the psoriatic plaques. When plaques are removed, punctuated bleeding can occur. This is called the Auspitz sign, and it can be explained by the infiltration of large blood vessels in the elongated *rete* ridge. Increased angiogenesis is also important in the disease's pathogenesis and is closely linked with the inflammation and leukocytes accumulation within the skin [27-28].

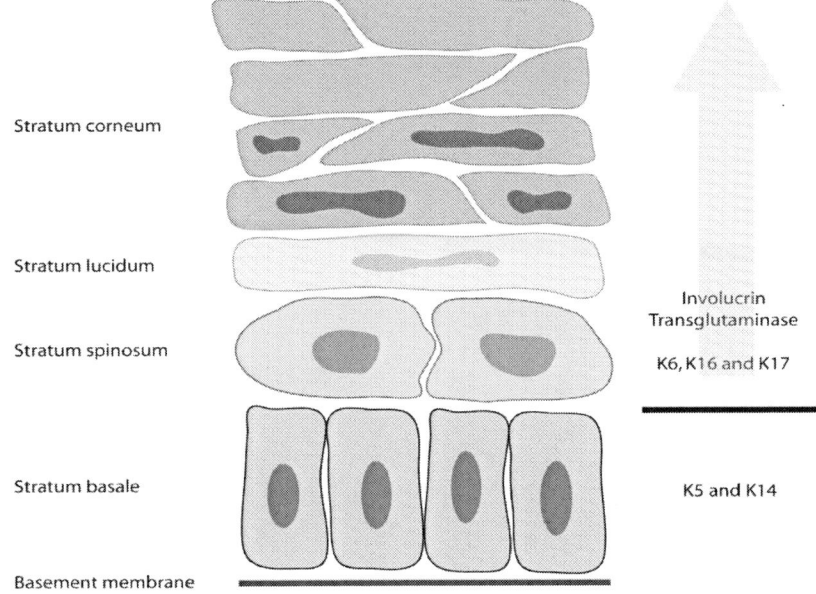

Figure 1. Schematic representation of the histological aspect of hyperproliferative psoriatic epidermis.

Chapter II

Causes of Psoriasis

Psoriasis is an inflammatory, multi-systemic skin disease characterized by hyperproliferation and abnormal differentiation of epidermis [23-24, 29-30]. Even if progress had been achieved in our comprehension of the pathogenesis of psoriasis, the exact cause is still unknown [31]. Today, four potential factors are suggested to be involved in the etiology of psoriasis: hyperproliferation and abnormal differentiation of the epidermis, oxidative stress, immune cells and genetics.

Hyperproliferation and Abnormal Differentiation of Psoriatic Keratinocytes

As previously mentioned, psoriasis is a hyperproliferative disease [32-33]. This hyperproliferation implies that psoriatic keratinocytes have a faster renewal than normal epidermis. In fact, psoriatic keratinocytes achieve the surface of the skin in 7 to 10 days, while, in the normal skin, the turnover process is about 28 to 50 days [34]. Pathological keratinocytes undergo the differentiation process more rapidly than normal keratinocytes and when they reach the surface of the skin, their maturation is incomplete [35].

The abnormal differentiation process brings many changes in the expression of cell-differentiation markers; especially for the keratins. Effectively, the basal keratins 5 and 14 are overexpressed in psoriasis [36]. However, other keratins, such as the suprabasal keratins 1 and 10, are underexpressed in psoriatic epidermis [37-38]. In psoriasis, these keratins are partially replaced by hyperproliferation ones: keratins 6, 16 and 17, well known in the literature to be expressed in hyperproliferative tissues such as psoriatic skins but absent in normal skins [39-41]. Enzymes and proteins involved in the formation of the *stratum corneum* (SC) are precociously expressed (Table 1; Figure 1). It is the case of transglutaminase and involucrin. Psoriatic skins also demonstrate a low expression of loricrin and filaggrin, which are normally expressed in the granular layer [42]. An exhaustive list of the differentiation markers and their expression in normal and psoriatic skins can be seen in Table 1.

Table 1. Expression of differentiation markers
in normal and psoriatic skins

Markers	Expression in normal skin	Expression in psoriatic skin	Ref
Epidermal			
Keratins 5 and 14	*Stratum basale*	Augmentation	[43]
Keratins 1 and 10	*Stratum suprabasale*	Reduction	[44]
Keratins 6, 16 and 17	Not expressed	*Stratum suprabasale*	[39-40]
Transglutaminase	Stratum spinosum	Augmentation and/or precocious	[45]
Involucrin	*Stratum spinosum*	Augmentation and/or precocious	[46]
Loricrin	*Stratum granulosum*	Totally or partially absent	[46]
Filaggrin	*Stratum granulosum*	Totally or partially absent	[36]
Dermo-epidermal			
Laminin	Basement membrane	Discontinued	[47]
Collagen VII	Basement membrane	Discontinued	[47]
Dermal			
Chondroitin sulfate	Upper dermis	Diffused	[48]
Collagen I	Dermis	Dermis	[49]
Fibronectin	Dermis	Dermis	[50]

Oxidative Stress in Psoriasis

A significant increase of scientific information supports the view that the skin's redox state is involved in skin disorders pathogenesis [51-52]. Skin functions as an interface between the body and the environment; it is chronically exposed to both endogenous and environmental oxidant agents, leading to generation of reactive oxygen species (ROS). Overproduction or an inadequate removal of ROS results in oxidative stress, leading to dysregulated signal transduction and pathological changes in cell and tissue functions [53].

In normal skin, keratinocytes are the major source of ROS, whereas in psoriatic skin, ROS are generated by both keratinocytes and activated neutrophils [54-55]. Psoriatic keratinocytes have a higher exposition to endogenous oxidants than those in normal skin. Additionally, psoriatic skin shows a defect in epidermal barrier function, which is a major pathophysiological factor [56]. Alterations in ceramide content and abnormal lipid organization of psoriatic *stratum corneum* are primarily involved in this reduced barrier function [57]. These alterations could be closely linked to lower skin defensive functions against external pro-oxidant agents, which is a critical factor driving a major skin exposition to environmental risk [58]. Altogether, these factors make psoriatic skin a tissue with abnormally high oxidative stress.

Studies on the implication of oxidative stress in psoriasis etiology mainly focused on establishing a correlation between antioxidant imbalance and oxidative damage. The results suggest a deficient antioxidant system, which could be a factor involved in the pathogenesis of psoriasis [59-60].

Psoriatic Blood Samples

Analyses of blood samples generally reveal lower concentration of low-molecular-weight antioxidants and antioxidant enzyme activities when compared with blood from normal donors [61-62] (Table 2). Erythrocytes' membranes from psoriatic patients have less vitamin E, selenium and glutathione [63]. Similarly, glutathione, selenium and β-carotene levels are reduced in psoriatic plasma [61-62].

Some studies show that psoriatic erythrocytes present no significant differences in catalase (CAT) activity [64-65], whereas most of reports show lower CAT activity as compared with normal erythrocytes [60, 66-67]. Higher glutathione peroxidase (GPx) activity in psoriatic erythrocytes has been determined by some studies [64, 67], whereas a majority of reports shows lower GPx activity when compared with healthy controls [60, 68-69]. With regard to superoxide dismutase (SOD) activity, the majority of reports shows that it is lower in psoriatic erythrocytes [60, 66-67], whereas others describe either no significant differences [65] or a higher SOD activity [64]. Lower and higher SOD activities have been reported in psoriatic plasma [60, 70].

Experimental evidence demonstrates that psoriatic blood samples display increased malondialdehyde levels, suggesting that psoriasis is associated with a lipid peroxidation status [68-69]. Lipid peroxidation products such as lipid hydroperoxide and autoantibodies against oxidized modified low-density lipoprotein have been found to be increased in psoriatic plasma [60]. Low-density lipoprotein oxidation and disturbances of oxidant-antioxidant balance have been associated with an increased risk for atherosclerosis in psoriatic patients [60]. In addition, increased nitric oxide (NO) levels from serum and plasma have been reported for psoriatic patients as compared with normal individuals [71-72].

Oxidative stress in blood samples seems to be linked with neutrophils activation and with psoriasis worsening [63]. Lactoferrin released by specific neutrophil granules promotes neutrophil-endothelial cell adhesion and, as a source of iron, the Fenton reaction, contributing to hydroxyl radical generation [63]. There is a positive correlation between neutrophils count in psoriatic blood with lipid peroxidation levels in plasma, which has been further correlated with lipid peroxidation in erythrocyte membranes [65]. Increase of erythrocyte lipid peroxidation correlates with decrease of membrane fluidity in these cells [73]. Plasma and erythrocyte oxidative damage have been further connected with psoriasis aggravation [65].

Psoriatic Skin

Skin proteins are vulnerable to oxidant damage. Consequently, protein carbonyl moieties are formed by both protein oxidative cleavage and amino acids direct oxidation. Levels of protein carbonylation in psoriatic fibroblasts and in biopsies of involved and uninvolved psoriatic skin are higher than in healthy controls (Table 2) [74]. In psoriatic skin, the activity of xanthine oxidase is higher [75], and the action of cytokines such as tumor necrosis factor alpha (TNF-α) can also contribute to ROS production [76].

Table 2. Antioxidants and oxidative markers in psoriasis

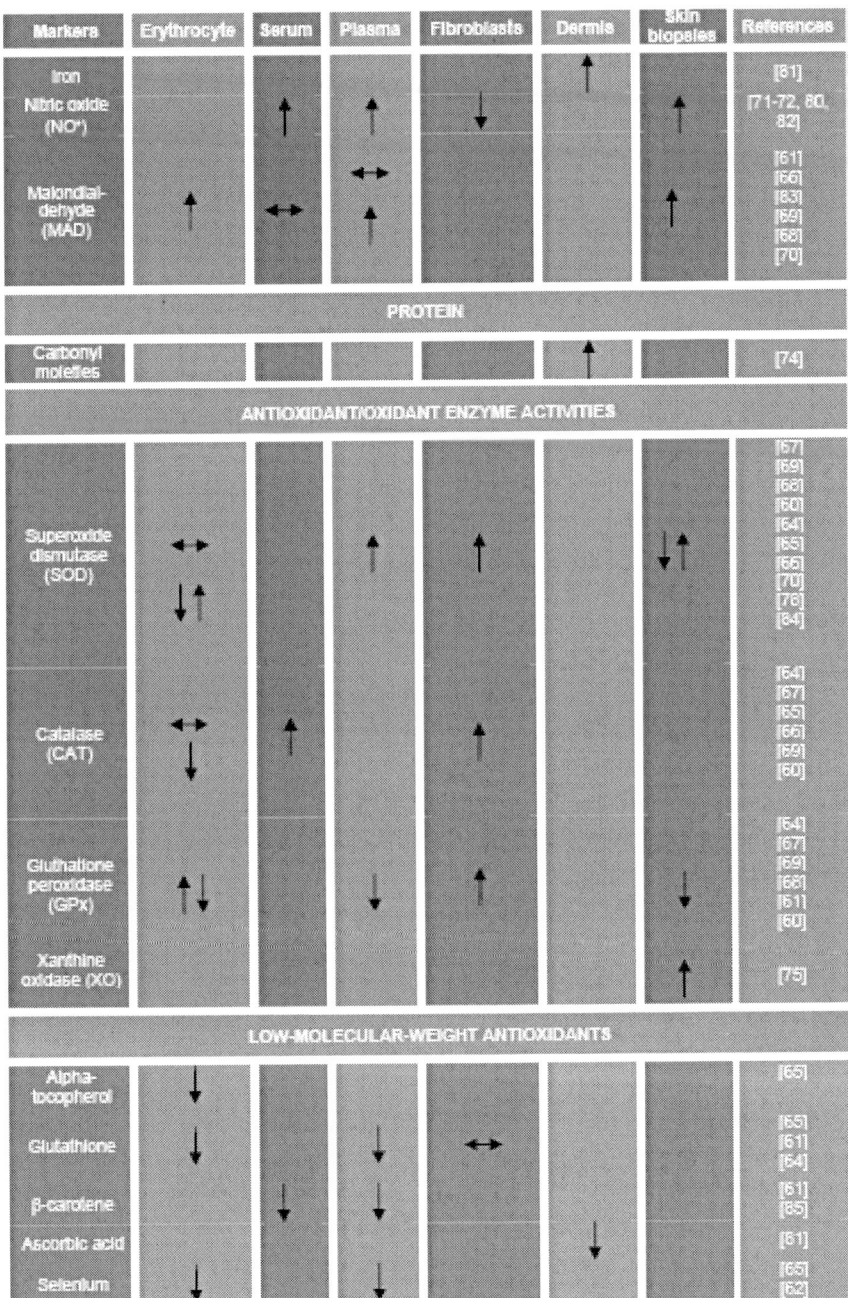

Antioxidant enzymes activities in psoriatic skin are often different as compared with psoriatic blood samples (Table 2). According to Therond et al., CAT activity was slightly enhanced in psoriatic fibroblasts from involved and uninvolved psoriatic skin, but GPx activity of involved and normal fibroblasts was not significantly different [64]. However, in tissues homogenates from psoriatic skin, GPx activity was found to be lower compared with those from normal skin [68]. Staining of frozen sections from normal and psoriatic skin with monoclonal antibodies against human CuZn-SOD and Mn-SOD showed that in psoriatic epidermis, Mn-SOD levels were considerably decreased [77]. In psoriatic tissue homogenates, SOD activity was also found to be lower as compared to those from normal skin [68]. However, significantly elevated CuZn-SOD activity in involved and uninvolved psoriatic skin and higher Mn-SOD activity in psoriatic fibroblasts have also been described [64]. MnSOD mRNA has also been reported to be markedly expressed in psoriatic skin lesions as compared with uninvolved psoriatic skin and normal controls [78]. Under normal conditions, Mn-SOD overexpression represents a protective cellular response evoked by both ROS and cytokines released interleukin (IL)-1β and TNF-α from inflammatory cells [78]. However, high or long-term SOD expression can also result in inappropriate production of hydrogen peroxide (H_2O_2) in intra- and extracellular compartments [79], contributing to inflammation and tissue damage at the site of psoriatic skin lesions [53].

In the context of psoriasis dermal vascular dilatation, NO role deserves special attention since it appears to be important for keratinocyte proliferation and angiogenesis [80]. Biopsies from involved and uninvolved psoriatic and normal skin were studied by immunochemistry in order to detect the presence of endothelial (eNOS), neuronal (nNOS) and inducible (iNOS) isoforms of nitric oxide synthase [80]. Endothelial nitric oxide synthase was not significantly expressed in psoriasis. However, iNOS was absent in normal skin but was significantly upregulated in involved psoriatic skin, mainly in keratinocytes and, to a lesser extent, in clinically uninvolved psoriatic skin [80]. Indeed, iNOS staining was greatest in the more severe lesions and correlated with the lymphoid infiltrate (CD3-positive cells) and also with keratinocyte proliferation. Measurement of NO production from the skin surface revealed a tenfold increase in the lesions of psoriatic patients compared with their uninvolved skin [80]. However, lack of significantly increased NO production by involved psoriatic fibroblasts as compared with healthy ones has also been reported [72].

Immunology of Psoriasis

The predominant role of immune cells in the pathogenesis of psoriasis is now well recognized [23, 86-88]. The importance of an abnormal T cells' activity in psoriasis is illustrated through both genetic predisposition and the mechanisms of action for a number of treatments. A complex interplay between keratinocytes, on one hand, and the cells of the innate and adaptive immune system along with a vast network of cytokines, on the other hand, produce an activation loop that leads to T cell activation, chronic inflammation within the skin and eventually the formation of psoriatic plaques. Immune cells included in this process, and found within active psoriatic plaques, are T cells (both CD4+ and CD8+), neutrophils, mast cells and dendritic cells [23]. Each has its own role and importance and will be further discussed through this section.

T Cells

T cells and the cytokines they secrete are the cornerstone of the immunological theory in psoriasis. The large amount of scientific information published provides a good understanding for the cascade of events leading to their activity in psoriatic plaques, including their initial activation and their migration in the skin.

Th1/Th2/Th17 Balance

For a long period of time, psoriasis was believed to be a T helper cell (Th)1-driven disease [89]. Th1 secretes interferon (IFN)-γ and TNF-α, both of which have been found in high concentration within psoriatic plaques and are known to have an important repercussion on keratinocytes. Indeed, they promote the expression of intercellular adhesion molecule 1 (ICAM-1) and human leukocyte antigen class II (HLA-DR) on keratinocytes surface [90-92]. ICAM-1 interacts and increases leukocyte adherence within the skin, whereas the expression of HLA-DR allows keratinocytes to present antigens to both CD4+ in addition to CD8+ T cells through MHC class I [90-92]. Thus, the Th1 pathway is important in the pathogenesis of the disease since it affects leukocytes recruitment and alters keratinocytes growth. However, recent investigations also demonstrated the importance of the Th17 pathway. Th17 are recently discovered CD4+ T cells that have also been associated with other inflammatory diseases such as asthma and Crohn's disease [93-95]. Th17 cells produce IL-17, a cytokine promoting production of IL-6, IL-8, GM-CSF, and ICAM-1 by keratinocytes, synergizing with the IFN-γ effect [93]. Such molecules will attract even more leukocytes within the skin. Also, these cells produce IL-22, a cytokine known to delay keratinocytes differentiation [96]. This new information is very important since it points to specific mechanisms.

The deviation of naive T cells into Th2 instead of Th1 or Th17 has proven to be an effective way to treat the disease, demonstrating the importance of the Th1/Th2/Th17 balance and the underlying mechanisms controlling this differentiation process. Induction of the Th1 pathway relies on IL-12, whereas the Th17 pathway relies on IL-6 and IL-23. The US Food and Drug Administration recently approved ustekinumab in the treatment of plaque psoriasis. This human monoclonal antibody targets IL-12p40, the common subunit of IL-12 and IL-23, hence reducing differentiation into Th17 [88, 97].

Even more recently, so-called Th22 were identified and linked to psoriasis [98-99]. This subset of Th cells were found to secrete a unique pattern of cytokines including IL-22 and TNF-α, similarly to Th17; while they do not secrete IFN-γ, IL-4 or IL-17, as opposed to Th1, Th2 and Th17 [98]. IL-22 is known, as mentioned above, to affect keratinocytes by promoting proliferation and inhibiting differentiation [98]. Thus, IL-22 seems to amplify TNF-α's effect in psoriatic plaques [98].

Although very important, T cells' activation is dependent of other cell types, such as dendritic cells. To understand the immunopathogenesis of psoriasis, the interaction of T cells with these other cell types is important because T cells are part of a complex pathological network.

Natural Killer T Cells

The role of natural killer T cells in psoriasis is not totally understood yet. This unique subpopulation of T cells expresses natural killer receptors (e.g., CD94 and CD161) and T cell receptors (e.g., CD4) on its surface, therefore combining proprieties of both lineages. They are considered to be an important part of the innate immunity, but they could also play an intermediary role between innate and adaptive immunity [100]. Natural killer T cells are another potential source of IFN-γ and TNF-α in psoriasis and can secrete cytokines implicated in the Th1 and Th2 balance (IL-2, IL-4, IL-5, IL-10, IL-13) [101]. Psoriatic keratinocytes express CD1d and can interact with CD161 of natural killer T cells [102]. This molecular interaction could be a critical event triggering the apparition of lesions in psoriasis, as CD1d is present in uninvolved skin of patients [101]. Also, the amount of CD4+CD161+ cells found in the skin is increased in psoriatic plaques and uninvolved skin as compared to normal subjects. Finally, various treatments were found to reduce the amount of CD94+ and CD161+ cells within the skin, including betamethasone dipropionate, calcipotriol and alefacept, suggesting an association between this decrease and clinical improvement [103-104].

Dendritic Cells

As mentioned earlier, a key event in T cells' activation is the presentation of antigens on the major histocompatibility complex (MHC) class II by antigens presenting cells such as dendritic cells [105-106]. Those cells also possess co-stimulatory molecules required by T cells to be activated. Such cells with the ability to present antigens and transmit co-stimulatory signals are known as professional antigens presenting cells and are fundamental in the activation loop of T cells. The most important co-stimulatory signals occur between CD28-CD80/CD86 and between CD40-CD154 [107] and could therefore be of interest as potential pharmacological targets [107].

In physiological conditions, dendritic cells will process antigens and then migrate to the lymph node where they can interact directly with T cells. Afterward, T cells activated by this antigen will proliferate within the lymph node, enter the systemic blood circulation, reach the tissue where the antigen was originally found and then exit the blood vessels. Local increases in the concentration of specific chemokines will guide T cells through most of the process. It has been proposed that in chronic psoriatic plaques, T cells and dendritic cells can form a lymphoid-type tissue in which the cellular interaction could happen directly within the skin, without going through the process of migration to the node and back to the inflammation site [89, 107-108]. Finally, dendritic cells secrete cytokines, such as IL-12, IL-15, IL-18, IL-23 and IFN-γ. Those cytokines promote Th1 and Th17 proliferation and are thus most likely involved in the Th1/Th2/Th17 balance [89].

Neutrophils

The role of neutrophils in psoriasis pathogenesis is not totally understood yet; its importance is therefore controversial. However, several facts suggest it could be essential in the early development of lesions [109]. For instance, a case report described rapid improvement of psoriasis lesions following an agranulocytosis induced by ticlopidine [110]. This report is particularly interesting because neutrophils' blood count correlated with a 24-hour delay, and symptoms reappeared in the days following blood count return to normal. The authors suggested a minimal number of neutrophils might be necessary in the early onset and the maintenance of psoriatic plaques [110]. Cytokines produced by T cells in psoriatic lesions induce the expression of the carcinoembryonic antigen-related cell adhesion molecule 1 (CEACAM1) on the surface of keratinocytes [111]. This protein is able to increase the lifespan of neutrophils and can therefore be responsible for the accumulation of neutrophils in the epidermis of psoriatic plaques, a histological hallmark known as microabcesses of Munro [111]. Also, the high concentration of IL-8 and GM-CSF found within psoriatic lesions can activate and increase neutrophils' lifespan within the skin. For their role in the pathogenesis of psoriasis, neutrophils seem to be effector cells, dependent on T cell cytokines, but, at the same time contribute to T cell activation through the expression of HLA-DR [112-113]. This activation loop could play an important role in the acute phase of psoriasis plaque's formation [109]. Neutrophils themselves could be partly responsible for tissue damage through oxidative stress caused by the release of ROS.

Finally, a decrease in the activity of gluthatione peroxidase in neutrophils isolated from psoriatic patients indicates it could also be, in part, responsible for the increased secretion of vascular endothelial growth factor (VEGF) by keratinocytes, since H_2O_2 is known to induce VEGF secretion and could thus indirectly promote angiogenesis [114].

Mast cells

Mast cells have long been known to play an essential role in allergic reaction through IgE binding. However, their role in other mechanisms of innate and adaptive immunity through the secretion of multiple soluble factors has only been discovered in the last decade [115]. In psoriatic plaques, there is an accumulation of mast cells [116]. It was demonstrated that interactions between mast cells and T cells result in the activation of different T cells subsets. This phenomenon could be important in the pathogenesis of psoriasis because of a preferential activation of the Th1/Th17 pathway rather than Th2 [117]. Mast cells also express MHC class II, allowing antigens presentation to CD4+ T cells. They were also shown to express CD80 and CD86 on their membrane, two co-stimulatory signals necessary for T cells' activation [115]. Finally, mast cells can rapidly secrete large amounts of cytokines that will attract a wide variety of immune cells seen in psoriasis such as T cells and neutrophils [115].

Cytokines

Throughout this section, a variety of cytokines and their respective roles toward specific immune cells were discussed. The vast pathological network of cytokines found in psoriasis links most cells in its complex pathogenesis [118].

Cytokines affect both the immune system activity while also interacting directly with skin cells such as keratinocytes to alter their proliferation, differentiation and their own secretion pattern [119-121]. A Th1/Th17 pattern is observed, in which both downstream (e.g., increased in TNF-α, IFN-γ and IL-17) and upstream products (e.g., increased in IL-12 and IL-23, decreased in IL-4 and IL-10) related to them are present in high concentrations within psoriatic plaques. Several chemokines, which attract leukocytes within the skin, are also found in high concentrations (e.g., MCP-1, RANTES, TARC, IL-8, IP-10) [119].

Genetics of Psoriasis

Psoriasis has long been known to have a strong inherited component; population studies demonstrated the increased incidence among relatives of psoriatic patients compared to the general population [122]. Those findings demonstrated the importance of heredity and the highly probable existence of susceptibility genes. However, psoriasis does not follow a simple monogenic mutation model. Major progress in the field of genetics in the past decades has allowed genome-wide mapping leading to several large-scale studies made in an attempt to understand the complex role of genetics in the disease [88]. Those studies were able to identify several susceptibility loci and, therefore, gave new insight to the disease itself. Genes identified from those loci mostly encode for immune system proteins such as MHC or for proteins found in the skin. This further confirms the complexity surrounding the etiology of the disease and the potential duality in its origins.

PSORS1

Of all susceptibility loci, the PSORS1 locus on 6p21 is by far the most important. It was identified in multiple large-scale genome-wide studies of a broad variety of populations [88, 123-128]. In contrast with other susceptibility loci for which contradictory results were often found in literature, PSORS1 is always identified as the most important. This can be explained by the much higher odds ratio conferred by this susceptibility locus compared to all others. This locus is, therefore, well established within the scientific community. It is estimated to account for 35 to 50% of the heritability of psoriasis [124]. Fine-mapping studies revealed a 300-kb region with at least 11 genes (including HLA-C, MICA, CDSN, HCR, PSORS1C3) [124]. Although several of these genes are biologically plausible candidates, many studies have identified HLA-Cw6 as the gene most likely responsible for the susceptibility in this region of the chromosome. This protein of the MHC I can trigger an immune response in psoriasis-like skin disorders, whereas only 55 to 60% of patients with psoriasis have this variant and about 10 to 15% of individuals without psoriasis carry it [129].

This could be explained either by the other PSORS discovered or by the complexity of PSORS1 itself. The difficulty in identifying the susceptibility gene in this locus is due to the extensive linkage disequilibrium observed within the MHC and the number of biological plausible candidates. For instance, some studies pointed out CDSN as another possible but less likely candidate gene of PSORS1 [124]. This gene encodes for corneodesmosin, a protein responsible for the cohesion of keratinocytes in the epidermis. This clearly demonstrated once again the complexity of the disease itself and the possible duality surrounding the primary defect leading to psoriasis. It is also very interesting to note that this locus is strongly associated with early onset psoriasis and to guttate psoriasis, which also usually occurs at a younger age [130]. On the other hand, late-onset of plaque psoriasis in patients over 50 years old does not seem to be associated with this locus [131].

Those variations in susceptibility genes could eventually lead to a new classification or new types of psoriasis based on etiology instead of phenotype only. This is important because it could affect recommended treatment since it could be adapted more specifically to the disease. This hypothetical situation in which genetic variants guide clinicians is known as pharmacogenomics, a growing discipline, which aims to personalize treatment based on genotypes instead of arbitrary recommendation.

PSORS2

Located at 17q25, contradictory results with this susceptibility locus have been published [132-135]. Most studies concentrated on the gene RAPTOR and the Runt-related transcription factor (RUNX)1 binding site between genes NAT9 and SLC9A3R1. SLC9A3R1 has a putative role in the formation of immune synapse [88]. It is also found in epidermis within the granular layer of normal skin [133]. Therefore, SLC9A3R is a biologically plausible candidate that could once again affect the immune system and the skin directly. However, as mentioned above, contradictory results were obtained by single nucleotide polymorphism (SNP) mapping between NAT9 and SCL9A3R1 genes and altering a RUNX1 binding site [132, 134-135]. This susceptibility locus was also associated with atopic dermatitis, but a SNP mapping study suggested psoriasis-related genes were not responsible for the association of this locus with atopic dermatitis [133].

PSORS4

This susceptibility locus is particularly interesting because it is located within the region of the epidermal differentiation complex on chromosome 1q21 [136]. Genes in this complex encode for proteins involved in the terminal differentiation of keratinocytes, a process deeply affected in psoriasis. Those proteins, such as filaggrin and loricrin, are essential in the cornification process. This susceptibility locus is, therefore, unique because, as opposed to most others, it could cause a defect directly within the skin differentiation process without affecting the immune system. Treatment effectiveness might be affected, and those patients might benefit from therapies that differ from the usual ones. Further research was able to identify that a deletion in genes of the late cornified envelope (LCE) 3B and 3C was responsible for this locus [137-140]. Although the mechanistic role of LCE in psoriasis remains to be understood, those proteins are important in the formation of the skin barrier and also its repair, two phenomena altered in psoriasis. Overlapping between atopic dermatitis and psoriasis was shown with the susceptibility locus in 1q21; however, it has been demonstrated that the genes within this locus do not display the same levels of influence for those two pathologies [141].

IL-12B

Along with IL-23R, they are the non-MHC susceptibility genes with the strongest association to psoriasis. IL-12B encodes for interleukin-12 beta sub-unit p40, which is also a sub-unit of IL-23. Many genome-wide studies revealed this susceptibility locus located in 5q31 [142-148]. Most studies reporting IL-12B as a susceptibility gene also found a strong association with IL-23R. This information is crucial since it identifies IL-23 and not IL-12 as an important cytokine in psoriasis. IL-23 promotes T cells' differentiation into Th17, a pathological pathway recently discovered and now believed to be of importance in the pathogenesis of psoriasis [93]. Ustekinumab, a recently approved biological treatment, is a human monoclonal anti-p40 antibody, which, therefore, aims to stop this preferential differentiation of T cells into Th17 [88, 149]. This proof of concept on the importance of IL-23, and the Th17 pathway also stresses the importance of genetic studies in psoriasis since it provides crucial information on core mechanisms behind the disease. Finally, this gene has also been associated with Crohn's disease, suggesting a possible common pathological pathway of inflammation shared in both pathologies [147, 150]. An association with atopic dermatitis has also been published, suggesting this IL-23 pathway could link many auto-immune diseases [146].

IL-23R

Located on chromosome 6p21, the identification of IL-23R as a risk factor of psoriasis supports the importance of the Th17 pathway mentioned above [142-147]. The concept of Th17 is relatively recent, but its role in auto-immune disease is now well established.

IL-4 and IL-13

The identification of the susceptibility locus on chromosome 5q31 in the cytokine gene cluster encoding for IL-4 and IL-13 also gave important information regarding the inflammatory pathway in psoriasis [142-143, 151-152]. As mentioned earlier, T cell differentiation is very important in the pathogenesis of psoriasis. The complex balance between Th1-Th2-Th17 is regulated by many cytokines, including IL-4 and IL-13. Those cytokines promote T cells' differentiation into Th2 and inhibit the differentiation of naïve T cells into Th1 and Th17 [153]. Low levels of both cytokines could, therefore, be responsible for an abnormal increase in Th1 and Th17 populations observed in psoriasis and other Th17 driven inflammatory disease. In fact, this gene cluster has also been associated with Crohn's disease; however, the variants are distinct for the two diseases [154].

Protein Tyrosine Phosphatase Nonreceptor Type 22 (PTPN22)

The PTPN22 gene encodes for the protein lymphoid tyrosine phosphatase, a molecule involved in T cell intracellular signaling [155]. This protein binds to CsK, a kinase that inhibits the Src family kinases. Therefore, PTPN22 exerts an inhibitory effect on T cells' receptor signalization. Susceptibility with this gene has been demonstrated by various research groups, but the association with psoriasis is not as strong as with other autoimmune diseases [156-158].

Indeed, polymorphism in PTPN22 has been clearly associated with many other auto-immune diseases, including Type 1 diabetes mellitus, juvenile idiopathic arthritis, systemic lupus erythematous, rheumatoid arthritis and autoimmune thyroid disease [88, 155]. However, the R620W polymorphism usually associated with those diseases is not a risk factor for psoriasis [158]. It is hypothesized that the mechanism underlying this very general susceptibility to auto-immunity associated with this gene is caused by an alteration in the positive selection of T cells in the thymus.

ZNF313

A 47 kb susceptibility locus located on chromosome 20q13 was discovered and associated with psoriasis [142, 159]. It was further demonstrated that the susceptibility gene was ZNF313 also known as RNF114. This protein is a member of RING domain E3 ubiquitin ligases [159]. Expressed by skin cells, T cells and dendritic cells, ZNF313 is a positive regulator of T cell activation. Protein ubiquitinylation regulates the immune response by modifying activity or promoting degradation of certain molecular signals and could, therefore, have an impact on T cells' activation within psoriatic plaques [160]. Members of this family have already been associated with other auto-immune diseases [161].

CDKAL1

The biological function of this gene is unknown but the transcript was shown to be almost absent from skin keratinocytes and abundant in CD4+ and CD19+ lymphocytes [162]. Therefore, it is difficult to discuss the significance of this susceptibility gene. However, it was shown to also give susceptibility to Crohn's disease [156, 162-163]. This gene is also associated with type II diabetes; however, this association is independent of the susceptibility observed for psoriasis and Crohn's disease [162]. It is interesting to note that this gene and others mentioned above confer susceptibility to Crohn's disease, which could partially explain the increased incidence of psoriasis observed in patients suffering from this disease. Those common susceptibility genes are all related to T cells, which once again demonstrate the cornerstone role played by these cells in the pathogenesis of psoriasis.

Chapter III

Treatments of Psoriasis

Generally, psoriasis is not a fatal disease, but the presence of physical and psychological pains can severely affect patients' quality of life [164]. There is a wide variety of therapeutic options to treat psoriasis, including topical, phototherapy, systemic and biological therapies (Table 3) [165]. These treatments can control or prevent symptoms; however, there is still no cure available [166-167]. Some treatments will be discussed in this section.

Table 3. Complete list of actual or future therapies for psoriasis

Topical	Phototherapy	Systemic	Biological
Corticosteroids	Broadband UVB	Methotrexate	Infliximab
Vitamin D analogues	Narrowband UVB	Acitretin	Etanercept
Tazarotene	Excimer Laser	Cyclosporine A	Adalimumab
Salicylic acid	Psoralen-UVA	Fumaric acid esters	Efalizumab
Calcineurin inhibitors		Sulfasalazine	Alefacept
		Hydroxyurea	Ustekinumab
		Mycophenolate mofetil	Briakinumab

Topical Treatments

Topical treatments are principally used to treat benign or moderate psoriasis. However, they can also be used to treat severe psoriasis if they are combined with systemic therapy [168-169]. Topical treatments can act on psoriasis in different ways: by reducing the local inflammation and/or the hyperproliferation of keratinocytes, by regulating the cell differentiation and finally, by re-establishing the integrity of the *stratum corneum* [170].

Corticosteroids

In 1952, hydrocortisone acetate, the first topical glucocorticoid developed for the treatment of inflammatory diseases, appeared on the market [171]. Since then, many corticosteroids had been developed to treat psoriasis. Today, topical corticosteroids are grouped according to their potency [170, 172]. They are the most widely prescribed topical treatment to treat psoriasis [173]. Their efficacy can be attributed to multiple mechanisms of action, including their anti-inflammatory, immunosuppressive and antiproliferative effects [174]. Corticosteroids bind to specific receptor proteins, and this complex interacts with specific DNA sequences, the glucocorticoid response elements, to regulate the expression of corticosteroid-responsive genes. This leads to a myriad of effects, including altered cytokine expression and T cells' inhibition [173]. Corticosteroids are also known to inhibit the transcription of pro-inflammatory cytokines genes involved in psoriasis such as the interleukins 1, 2 and 6, while they can stimulate the expression of anti-inflammatory cytokines genes such as interleukin 10 [174]. Corticosteroids are quite effective to treat psoriasis. However, their combination with some substances can boost their potency [168]. For example, the combination of corticosteroids with salicylic acid, which possesses keratolytic properties, enhances penetration of the treatment [175]. The use of corticosteroids is safe, but the prolonged use is limited by tachyphylaxis and various side effects [165, 173].

Vitamin D Analogues

Many vitamin D analogues have been developed for the treatment of psoriasis. Calcipotriol and calcitriol are the only vitamin D analogues approved in the United States [176-177]; tacalcitolis is only available in

Europe [176]. They are of interest in the treatment of psoriasis because they can regulate the hyperproliferation and the abnormal differentiation of psoriatic keratinocytes [170]. Vitamin D analogues bind the vitamin D receptor, which binds to vitamin D response elements. This interaction leads to the alteration in the transcription of vitamin D responsive genes, resulting in the inhibition of keratinocyte proliferation and the stimulation of keratinocyte differentiation. Topical calcitriol also decreases intercellular adhesion molecule ICAM-1 expression on keratinocytes and T cells' infiltration [173]. Calcitriol is very efficient with minimal side effects, but the results are only apparent after a long period of use.

Tazarotene

Tazarotene is an acetylate retinoid derived from the synthesis of vitamin A [170], which is rapidly metabolized to its active metabolite: tazarotenic acid [173]. It is recognized for its role as a regulator of cell proliferation and differentiation via an interaction with the RAR-γ receptor [178]. Three genes seem to be affected by the tazarotenic acid, namely TIG1, TIG2 and TIG3. Tazarotene modulates the pathogenesis of psoriasis through three mechanisms: (1) reduction in keratinocyte proliferation, (2) normalization of keratinocyte differentiation and (3) a decrease in the expression of inflammatory mediators [173-174]. In an indirect way, tazarotenic acid seems to form a complex with the RAR-γ receptor, which would reduce the quantity of AP-1, a protein present in hyperproliferative skin disorders such as psoriasis [174]. However, this mechanism is not well known. Tazarotene also regulates many markers of cell differentiation, which are overexpressed (transglutaminase, keratins 6 and 16 and involucrin) or underexpressed (keratin 10 and filaggrin) in psoriasis [179]. Because this treatment has an important inflammatory potential, it is more effective when it is combined with topical corticosteroids [168, 180]. Tazarotene is the only topical retinoid used to treat psoriasis [168-169]. Some local side effects can be observed after the treatment, such as cutaneous irritation, burning sensations, itch and erythema [173]. That could explain the lack of use of this treatment in inverse psoriasis.

Salicylic Acid

The salicylic acid structure was first identified in 1838. It is the most ancient substance, which possesses a keratolytic effect [175]. Salicylic acid is generally combined with topical corticosteroids to enhance penetration [173]. This substance acts by increasing the permeability of the epidermis. Salicylic acid reduces the cohesion of the *stratum corneum,* by dissolving intercellular lipids and by reducing its pH, thereby increasing the hydration of the skin [170, 173]. Salicylic acid used alone helps decrease the quantity of plaques. In psoriasis, this substance is usually prescribed in combination with other treatments such as corticosteroids. It allows them to penetrate more quickly through the skin and to accelerate their action and their efficiency. Moreover, a study on the penetration of topical corticosteroids in the presence of salicylic acid showed that the active molecules had penetrated between two and three times more quickly [175]. However, because of the irritating character of salicylic acid, it is better to avoid its combination with vitamin D analogues [168]. Although salicylic acid is considered a secure treatment, side effects can be observed. For example, there is a risk of toxicity if the application takes place on more than 20% of the body, with symptoms such as nausea and hyperventilation [170, 181]. It is also important to note that salicylic acid can degrade some corticosteroids and make them inactive [181].

Tar

For many years, tar preparations have been used in the treatment of psoriasis for their antipsoriatic effects [182]. Tar is normally used in the form of shampoos and bath oils. However, the unpleasant smell makes it an unpopular treatment [178]. The mechanism is not completely characterized, but it includes antiproliferative, antipruritic, and antibacterial effects [173, 183].

Phototherapy

There are two types of phototherapy: the phototherapy UVB (broadband, narrowband and excimer laser) and the PUVA-therapy (oral or local). Mechanisms of action of both UVA and UVB phototherapy differed, but they achieve similar efficacy [184]. The main effects of UV irradiation on keratinocytes are the induction of apoptosis, inhibition of antigen presentation and the expression of immunosuppressive cytokines [185]. Phototherapy is often used when psoriasis cannot be controlled by topical treatments [186].

Phototherapy UVB

In broadband-UVB phototherapy, the skin is exposed to ultraviolet light from 290 to 320 nm [187]. Narrowband-UVB emits a distinct narrow band of high-intensity light from 311 to 313 nm. Narrowband-UVB shows a superior efficacy, compared to broadband-UVB, with fewer side effects. This helps eliminate high-energy shorter wavelengths responsible for burning, premature aging and increased incidence of skin cancer [186]. Because of its efficacy and its short-term tolerance, it tends to replace conventional phototherapy [168]. The principle of UVB phototherapy is based on the use of solar-type radiation to induce DNA damage and inactivate various proteins, resulting in antimitotic, anti-inflammatory and immunosuppressive effects. After a UVB phototherapy treatment, there is a reduction of IFN-γ, IL-2 and TNF-α levels in psoriatic patients [188].

Excimer Laser

The 308 nm excimer laser has documented clinical results that appear superior to broadband- and narrowband-UVB phototherapy with low accumulation of UVB doses [189]. However, laser treatment can only be used on small areas, because of the localized action of the laser itself. The exact mechanism of action is not completely known. However, it is suggested that the excimer laser penetrates the epidermis and the dermis to cause T cell apoptosis, whereas traditional UVB appears to induce T cell apoptosis only in the epidermis [189]. Laser therapy may be useful for the treatment of more resistant psoriatic lesions [168]. Furthermore, side effects that include erythema, burns and hyperpigmentation are limited to localized areas in contrast to larger areas seen with full-body treatments using traditional phototherapy [186].

Phototherapy UVA

PUVA-therapy consists of using a photosensitizing medication taken orally or absorbed topically in combination with UVA phototherapy (320 to 400 nm) [186]. The administration of psoralen by oral route, before the irradiation, allows the absorption of UVA radiations and the appearance of an antipsoriatic effect [183-184]. Once the psoralen is activated by light, it binds to DNA, prevents the replication of keratinocytes, and leads to the apoptosis of T cells in the skin [190]. Due to its cumulative toxicity, the PUVA-therapy is used as a first-line treatment in combination with other treatments such as tazarotene and acitretin [178]. Numerous side effects can be noted, including nausea, vomiting, itching and cancer [181], but remission can be observed in 80% of cases [190]. To encounter the unwanted effects caused by the oral administration, baths of psoralen, consisting of immersing parts of the body in a bath containing psoralen and exposing the patient to UVA, can be used [191]. Nevertheless, the PUVA-therapy tends to be replaced by the phototherapy UVB because of its numerous severe side effects [168, 183].

Systemic Treatments

Methotrexate

Methotrexate has been used to treat psoriasis for more than 40 years [192]. At the beginning, studies suggested that methotrexate acted directly against the keratinocyte hyperproliferation [193], however, the ineffectiveness of locally administrated methotrexate, as well as the effectiveness of immunosuppressive therapy, strongly suggest that the anti-proliferative effect of this treatment was not responsible of the anti-psoriatic effect [194]. In 2005, Johnston et al. reported that the effectiveness of methotrexate in psoriasis was due to anti-inflammatory mechanisms (suppression of T cells' activation and T cells' adhesion molecules expression mediated by adenosine or polyglutamated methotrexate) rather than apoptosis. Furthermore, methotrexate is also known to be a competitive inhibitor of the dihydrofolate reductase enzyme, which is essential for the DNA synthesis, thus leading to a decreased cell proliferation in psoriatic keratinocytes [187]. Although methotrexate treatment is efficient, many severe side effects can be observed, such as hepatic toxicity, pneumonia and teratogenicity [169].

Retinoids

Retinoids are derived from vitamin A and are widely used for the treatment of skin disease. Acitretin is an oral aromatic retinoid approved for the treatment of psoriasis [195]. It acts as an anti-proliferative and anti-inflammatory agent on psoriatic keratinocytes [192]. Although the complete mechanism is still unknown, it has been demonstrated that acitretin acts by activating the three retinoic acid receptors, which bind to nuclear response elements in genes controlling cell proliferation and differentiation, anti-inflammation, anti-keratinization and inhibition of neutrophil chemotaxis [196]. In this case, the use of combination therapy, rather than monotherapy, can be beneficial in increasing efficacy while reducing toxicity [183]. Acitretin is not well tolerated in high doses, and several side effects such as hepatic toxicity, teratogenicity and hyperlipidemia can be observed [187].

Cyclosporine

Cyclosporine is an anti-inflammatory agent, which allows the disappearance of psoriatic plaques [188]. Its mechanism of action implies the inhibition of calcineurin phosphatase, which prevents the transcription of genes involved in T lymphocyte activation and those regulating cytokines such as IL-2 and IL-4 [187-188]. Furthermore, cyclosporine also blocks proliferating keratinocytes in their G1 phase [197]. The important side effects associated with a cyclosporine treatment (renal toxicity and high blood pressure) restrict its use over a prolonged period of time [187, 192]. Effectively, cyclosporine is rather used as first-line treatment to remove plaques and is then replaced by a maintenance treatment with fewer side effects [192].

Biological Treatments

Biological therapies provide immunologically directed intervention when systemic treatments fail [198]. Biological agents are defined as fusion (or recombinant) proteins or monoclonal antibodies that possess pharmacological activity [199]. They can act by (1) reducing pathogenic T cells, (2) inhibiting T cell activation, (3) leading to an immune deviation or (4) blocking the activity of inflammatory cytokines involved in psoriasis [198].

Infliximab

Infliximab is an anti-TNF-α monoclonal IgG1 antibody [200], which acts in psoriasis by blocking TNF-α and by inhibiting the production of pro-inflammatory cytokines, the infiltration of inflammatory cells and the proliferation of keratinocytes [198]. Infliximab is associated with rapid and significant improvement of psoriatic lesions, but also with severe potential adverse effects. For example, infliximab treatment can cause anaphylactic shocks, cardiac insufficiencies, fungal infections and neurological problems [181, 201].

Etanercept

Etanercept is a TNF-receptor fusion protein produced by the fusion of two TNF receptors and the Fc fragment of human immunoglobulin (IgG1) [202]. Etanercept binds to TNF-α with a greater affinity than natural monomeric receptors [198]. TNF-α, which is bound by etanercept, is biologically inactive, resulting in reduced inflammation [202]. Etanercept has fewer side effects than other anti-TNF-α agents [203]. Among these side effects: flu-like symptoms and cardiac insufficiency [181].

Adalimumab

Adalimumab, another TNF-α blocker, is a completely humanized monoclonal, IgG1 antibody against TNF-α. Similar to infliximab, adalimumab binds strongly to soluble and transmembrane TNF-α, thereby preventing them from binding with their receptors. Adalimumab brings many side effects such as reactions to the injection site, increased risk of contracting a severe infection, immunosuppression of the bone marrow and increased incidence of tumors [204].

Efalizumab

Efalizumab is a recombinant humanized IgG1 monoclonal that binds and blocks CD11a [202]. This molecule, as well as CD18, is a subunit of the lymphocyte function-associated antigen 1 (LFA-1), which is an important surface molecule for T cells' activation, their migration inside the skin, and their cytotoxic function. The binding of efalizumab to CD11a blocks the interaction between LFA-1 and ICAM-1 [205]. In June 2009, after the appearance of severe bacteriological, viral, and fungal infections of some patients, Genentech decided to remove its product from the market.

Alefecept

Alefacept is a human fusion protein that consists of the extracellular CD2-binding portion of the human leukocyte functioning antigen 3 (LFA-3) linked to the Fc (hinge, CH2 and CH3 domains) fragment of human IgG1. It selectively blocks the LFA-3:CD2 costimulatory pathway, which is important in the reactivation of memory effector T cells. [206]. Alefacept also binds to CD2 on memory-effector T cells and prevents the generation of signal 2 [200, 207]. This connection triggers apoptosis in lymphocytes T of type CD4+, CD8+ and CD45RO+, which are highly expressed in psoriatic plaques [198, 208]. The side effects can include flu-like symptoms, reactions at the site of injection, tumors and infections [165].

Ustekinumab and Briakinumab

New biological treatments recently appeared on the market: ustekinumab and briakinumab (ABT-874). Comprehension of the mechanisms of action is still incomplete, but it is known that the antibody decreased the biological activity of interleukins 12 and 13 and reduced the inflammation [209].

Ustekinumab was approved in Europe and in Canada in 2008, and more recently in United States. Briakinumab is still undergoing Phase III trials, but preliminary results are interesting [88, 97, 209]. The main side effects are the presence of reactions at the site of injection and an increased incidence for some infections [200, 209].

Chapter IV

Pathological Models of Psoriasis

For the past decade, many pathological models have been developed to have a better understanding of psoriasis and to find out its exact cause [210-211]. The development of these models represents a key component for the fight against psoriasis. Applying research upon further development of these models represents key artillery for the battle against psoriasis disease.

In Vivo Models

Spontaneous Mutations

Psoriasis is a typical human skin disease. Instead, literature shows many cases of spontaneous mutations demonstrating psoriasis-like phenotype in mice [212], some of which were studied for their psoriasis-like characteristics, such as skin thickening and plaques formation [213]. However, the resulting rodent mutants do not mimic the human disease closely enough to be considered good models of psoriasis. These mutants must rather be used to compare local pathogenic events such as hyperkeratosis [213-215]. Among hundreds of listed mutations, three models were preferred. First, the *asebia* mouse mutation ($Scd1^{ab}/Scd1^{ab}$), characterized by an acanthosis, increased dermal vascularization, and dermal infiltrate comprising macrophages and mast cells, although neither T cells nor neutrophils were reported to be found [214-215]. This model is poorly representative of the human pathology in a way that it possesses no other characteristic of the disease, besides showing alterations of the cutaneous lipid metabolism, which seem to be different from what is usually observed on actual human psoriatic skin. The two other models are the spontaneous chronic proliferative dermatitis and the flaky skin mice (Ttc^{fsn}/Ttc^{fsn}). They show characteristics found in psoriasis such as hyperproliferative skin, infiltration of inflammatory cells in the skin, and dilation of blood vessels in the dermis. However, the absence of reaction after an immunosuppressive therapy suggests that these models are still incomplete; therefore, it appears uncertain to use such animal models for testing of potentially new therapeutic compounds [216-217].

Xenotransplantation

Xenotransplantation consists of transplanting on a genetically modified mouse a piece of psoriatic skin coming from a patient or, alternatively, a skin equivalent produced in laboratory. Many models based on immunodeficient mice have been developed in laboratories to study psoriasis disease. Among these models, we indicate the use of athymic nude mice [218-219], severe combined immunodeficient mice (SCID) [220] and the spontaneous AGR129 model [221].

The main difference between each model is the immunological potential of the immune system. Indeed, athymic nude mice have no thymus and, therefore, no T cells [220], while the severe combined immunodeficient mouse model lacks both T and B cells, yet displays functional neutrophil and mature natural killer (NK) cells with normal activity [210]. Finally, the AGR129 mice also lack both T and B cells, but, unlike of the severe combined immunodeficient mice, they still have immature NK cells, which are less cytotoxic than mature NK cells [221].

A weaker immune system is potent to dwell skin transplants for a longer time on a compromised mouse upon rejection. Thus, the amount of transplant rejection is reduced in the AGR129 model compared to the others. Boyman et al. demonstrated that human uninvolved psoriatic skin grafted onto AGR129 mice spontaneously developed psoriatic plaques without the injection of any activated immune cells or any other exogenous factor. In fact, skin grafts developed a psoriatic phenotype in 28 out of 31 (90%) grafted mice [210]. These results suggest that uninvolved psoriatic skin is not exactly comparable to normal skin from a healthy patient [217].

Genetically Engineered Models

The development of transgenic and knockout models for rats and for mice was an important step forward in the field of *in vivo* models. These genetically modified animals allow the overexpression or underexpression of a particular cytokine- or enzyme-creating rodent with psoriasis-like characteristics [222-224]. Currently, transgenic animal models only allow studying a single gene at a time. Since psoriasis is a multifactorial disease, models involving transgenic rodents are thus incomplete and do not allow the complete understanding of all of the histological and physiological characteristics of psoriasis. Genetically engineered mice represent the largest category of *in vivo* psoriasis models. The complete list of these *in vivo* models of psoriasis is presented in Table 4.

Table 4. Genetically engineered *in vivo* models of psoriasis. Modified from Jean et al., 2010 [217]

Model	Epidermal thickness	Abnormal differentiation	Increased vascularization	Epidermal T cell infiltration	References
Targeting the immune system					
HLA-B27/β2 microglobulin rat	+	+	+	+	[224-225]
Hypomorphic CD18	+	+	+	+	[222, 226]
αE (CD103)	+	+	?	+	[227]
K14/p40	+	?	?	+	[228]
Targeting vascular endothelium					
pTek-*tTA*/Tie2	+	+	+	+	[229]
K14/VEGF	+	+	+	+	[230]
Targeting epidermal proteins					
K5/Stat3C	+	+	+	+	[231]
IKK2	+	+	?	-	[232]
c-Jun/JunB	+	+	+	+	[233]
K14/KGF	+	+	+	-	[234]
K14/TGF-α	+	+	?	Some animals	[235]
K14/IL-20	+	+	-	-	[236]

Table 4. (Continued).

Model	Epidermal thickness	Abnormal differentiation	Increased vascularization	Epidermal T cell infiltration	References
K14/amphiregulin	+	+	+	+	[237]
K14/IL-1α	+	+	-	?	[238]
K14/IL-6	+	-	-	-	[239]
K10/BMP-6	+	+	+	+	[240]
Involucrin/integrins	+	+	+	+	[241]
Involucrin/MEK1	+	+	?	+	[242]
Involucrin/amphiregulin	+	+	+	+	[243]
Involucrin/IFN-γ	+	+	+	-	[244]
Chymotryptic enzyme	+	+	?	+	[245]

In Vitro Models

In vitro models offer an interesting alternative to animal models. Although inflammatory cells can be introduced in many *in vitro* skin models, they generally lack this element. Since inflammatory cells have been described to play a role in the pathogenesis of psoriasis [23-24, 29-30], the pertinence of these models has been questioned. However, recent studies using animal models, including the IKK2 [232] and c-Jun/JunB transgenic mice [233] are challenging the immunological theory of psoriasis [217].

Monolayer

The use of monolayer models has many advantages. First, the harvesting of a small biopsy of pathological skin (6 mm) allows the obtainment of a sufficient number of cells to conduct hundreds of experiments. Second, the monolayer offers the advantage of isolating each different cell type to better understand their specific roles and to dissect step by step the pathological mechanisms. On the other hand, because of the absence of interaction between dermis and epidermis or the frequent absence of inflammatory cells, these models are often considered as "incomplete". However, regardless of those limitations, studies using monolayer models have brought important advances in the current understanding of psoriasis [217].

Collagen Gel

Organ Culture

A way to rapidly obtain a three-dimensional model of psoriasis refers to the organ culture technique, which consists of putting a small biopsy of pathological skin on a collagen gel equivalent [246]. In this model, cell proliferation can be estimated by measuring the total surface area covered by the keratinocytes over a precise period of time. In 1985, Saiag et al. showed that higher keratinocyte proliferation rates were observed in the presence of psoriatic fibroblasts compared to keratinocytes cultured with normal fibroblasts [246]. They also demonstrated that normal fibroblasts are unable to suppress the hyperproliferation of psoriatic keratinocytes [217, 246].

Models Using Many Cellular Types

In order to obtain a more suitable model for studies about interactions between fibroblasts and keratinocytes, models using many cell types have been developed. In these models, fibroblasts, extracted from a normal or a psoriatic biopsy, are embedded in a collagen gel to form a dermis, whereas keratinocytes are seeded on the top of this dermal equivalent to generate the epidermis. In 1996, Konstantinova et al. developed a psoriatic skin model on a collagen gel, which highlighted many characteristics of psoriasis [247]. Their work yielded a number of interesting observations, such as the occurrence of a higher concentration rate in the secretion of IL-8 from uninvolved and involved psoriatic fibroblasts compared to normal fibroblasts [247]. In 2004, Barker et al. developed another psoriatic model on collagen gel. Their model maintained many characteristics of *in vivo* psoriatic skin such as hyperproliferation, overexpression of chemokine receptor CXCR2, pro-inflammatory genes (TNF-α, INF-γ and IL-8) and increased levels of pro-inflammatory cytokines IL-6 and IL-8 [248]. Like IKK2 [232] and c-Jun/JunB transgenic mice models [233], this model suggested that, even in the absence of T cells, pathological individuals possess an inherent predisposition of developing psoriasis characteristics [248]. The Konstantinova and Barker models are produced with different cell types, which allow different kinds of observation of interactions between dermal and epidermal cells; however, the presence of exogenous material still remains. Even if collagen gel can be quite useful for rapid production of three-dimensional models [249-251], the presence of an exogenous scaffold can be disadvantageous for mechanical studies of the extracellular matrix as well as for surface area studies, which could be reduced by retraction following collagen contraction of dermal substitutes [217, 252-253].

Self-Assembly Model

The self-assembly method allows the observation of interactions between fibroblasts and keratinocytes without any exogenous scaffold. Within this method, normal or pathological fibroblasts are cultured over a period of 28 days with ascorbic acid. Meanwhile, fibroblasts proliferate and secrete their own extracellular matrix to form dermal sheets in the flasks. After the 28-day period, two manipulatable sheets are superimposed and incubated for seven days to generate the dermal component. One week later, keratinocytes are seeded on top of the dermis to form a new epidermis. After another seven days of culture, the substitutes are lifted to the air–liquid interface to facilitate epidermal cell differentiation (Figure 2) [254-255].

In 2009, Jean et al. demonstrated that this model keeps many characteristics observed in psoriatic skins *in vitro* such as thickening of epidermis, the absence of a granular layer, hyperproliferation and abnormal differentiation of keratinocytes [256]. Furthermore, Bernard et al. demonstrated a disorganization of SC lipids such as those observed in psoriatic skin *in vivo* [257]. These results suggest that the self-assembly method allows the production of *in vitro* psoriatic skin models, which maintain a large number of psoriatic characteristics without any exogenous material or even T cells.

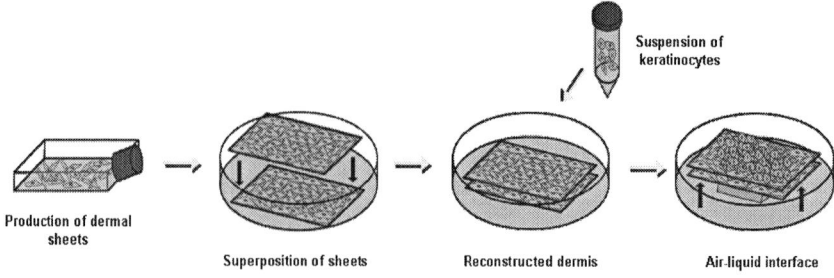

Figure 2. Self-assembly method. Modified from Jean et al., 2010 [217].

Chapter V

Advances of Concepts on the Pathogenesis of Psoriasis

The progress of concepts on the pathogenesis of psoriasis has been linked to the translation of clinical observations to basic scientific investigation. At the same time, the pathogenesis of this disease has been studied in laboratory models and subsequently translated to clinical experience in humans [258]. Given the absence of an accepted model to study psoriasis, many rounds of bidirectional translation (from clinical experience to laboratory investigation and *vice versa*) have taken place in order to better define its pathogenesis and find new treatments [258].

Many hypotheses have been proposed to explain the pathogenesis of psoriasis, such as an abnormal function of keratinocytes, dermal fibroblasts, vascular growth and immune cells [259-261]. In 1925, Goeckerman introduced phototherapy in combination with crude coal tar for psoriasis treatment [262]. Interestingly, this highly effective therapy for psoriasis was developed without any understanding of its pharmacological mechanism [258]. In 1951, Gubner described a series of psoriatic patients who were treated with aminopterin, a therapeutic approach based on the property of this agent to target hypermetabolic epithelial tissues like psoriatic epidermis [263]. Subsequently, methotrexate, an inhibitor of the enzyme dihydrofolate reductase and related to aminopterin, was used as an antagonist of keratinocyte hyperplasia with the idea that it would target the proliferation of involved psoriatic keratinocytes [264]. The successful therapeutic use of methotrexate inspired a flurry of clinical and laboratory research on aberrant psoriatic keratinocyte growth and differentiation [258]. Thus, rapid cell cycling and maturation of psoriatic keratinocytes as compared with normal keratinocytes were established as hallmarks of this skin disease [265]. In addition, the aberrant differentiation in psoriasis was described to be similar to regenerative maturation in skin wounds [266]. In 1982, Braverman and Sibley demonstrated that vascular proliferation was associated with epidermal hyperplasia in psoriasis [267].

In 1983, Bos and colleagues applied monoclonal antibodies to the detection of leukocyte subsets in psoriatic lesions [268]. Thus, they were the first to propose a potential role of the cellular immune system in the pathogenesis of psoriasis [258]. T cell differentiation was later found to be strongly polarized towards the type 1 pathway, with production of the cytokines such as IFN-γ and TNF-α [269]. During the 1980s, two hypotheses were proposed for psoriasis pathogenesis, one related to keratinocyte activation as a primary defect and another to the primary role of cellular immunity [258]. As activated keratinocytes were shown to produce many immune-activating cytokines [270], the cellular immune infiltration/activation was explained from the keratinocytes defect. However, a strong argument for psoriasis as a T cell-mediated autoimmune disease came from the treatment with cyclosporine, since it caused a significant improvement in the appearance of psoriatic lesions [271]. The T cell hypothesis for psoriasis pathogenesis was further supported by two approaches: in one, uninvolved psoriatic skin was grafted to SCID mice and shown to maintain a normal appearance. Further injection of activated mononuclear leucocytes into the grafts caused conversion to active psoriatic plaques [272]. Secondly, therapy with targeted immune antagonists such as a fusion protein with specific cellular toxicity to cells expressing functional IL-2 receptors confirmed the direct link between T lymphocytes and psoriasis. Thus, patients treated with deneleukin difitox, which did not specifically affect keratinocytes, exhibited clinical resolution of psoriasis with histological reversal of epidermal hyperplasia [273]. The utilization of the CTLA4-Ig fusion protein reduced the infiltration of activated T cells and dendritic cells (DCs) in psoriatic plaques, thereby resulting in clinical and pathological disease reversal in psoriatic patients [274-275]. The reduction of DCs infiltration following this treatment was very important since it conferred an important role for proteins expressed on activated DCs as potential targets in psoriasis [269].

The logical extension of immune targeting of psoriasis led to the development of new biological therapies [258]. Biological agents target specific molecules implied in psoriasis pathogenesis. So far, these fall into two main groups, targeting either specific inflammatory mediators such as TNF-α or T cells [23]. The response of psoriasis to TNF-α inhibitors suggested that this cytokine had a key role in psoriasis pathogenesis. TNF-α has complex interactions to support inflammation as well as regulate T cells and DCs interactions in the skin [276]. In addition, TNF-α shows effects on tissue remodeling, cell motility, cell cycle, and apoptosis [277-278]. Although biological treatments targeting TNF-α cytokine are highly effective in psoriasis, the elimination of TNF^+ leucocytes could suppress normal immune reactions that are not strictly TNF-dependent, thereby affecting protective immune responses during a lifetime of the treatment [23].

Overall, rapid advances in our understanding of psoriasis have occurred over recent years, thereby changing the concepts of psoriasis pathogenesis. Thus, psoriasis is now viewed as a process driven by an orchestrated interplay between activated T cells, antigen-presenting cells, and keratinocytes [23, 269], which leads to the release of numerous cytokines and chemokines that signal keratinocytes to hyperproliferate and undergo abnormal differentiation [279].

Chapter VI

Conclusion

The prevalence of psoriasis in the world is not negligible, and even if psoriasis is generally not a fatal disease, the consequences of this pathology on patients' quality of life are important. The development of new treatments has reduced many of the symptoms, allowing control of psoriasis and to ameliorate the quality of life of psoriatic patients; however, there is still no cure for this disease. The apparition of pathological skin models has facilitated the evolution of concepts, resulting in a better comprehension of this complex skin disease and in the development of more specific treatments with fewer side effects.

Acknowledgements

The authors gratefully thank Dr. Dan Lacroix and Jean-François Côté for the revision of the book.

References

[1] Meenan, F.O. A note on the history of psoriasis. *Ir. J. Med. Sci.,* 1955 6, 141-142.

[2] Glickman, F.S. Lepra, psora, psoriasis. *J. Am. Acad Dermatol.,* 1986 14, 863-866.

[3] Christophers, E. Psoriasis—epidemiology and clinical spectrum. *Clin. Exp. Dermatol.,* 2001 26, 314-320.

[4] Duffy, D.L.; Spelman, L.S. and Martin, N.G. Psoriasis in Australian twins. *J. Am. Acad. Dermatol.,* 1993 29, 428-434.

[5] Braathen, L.R.; Botten, G. and Bjerkedal, T. Prevalence of psoriasis in Norway. *Acta Derm. Venereol. Suppl.* (Stockh), 1989 142, 5-8.

[6] Neimann, A.L.P., SB; Gelfand, J.M. The epidemiology of psoriasis. *Expert. Rev. Dermatol.,* 2006 1, 63-75.

[7] Farber E.M. and ML, N. *Psoriasis Epidemiology: Natural history and genetics.* New York: Roenigk HH, MH; 1998; 107-158.

[8] Gelfand, J.M., et al. The prevalence of psoriasis in African Americans: results from a population-based study. *J. Am. Acad. Dermatol.,* 2005 52, 23-26.

[9] Naldi, L. Epidemiology of psoriasis. *Curr. Drug Targets Inflamm Allergy,* 2004 3, 121-128.

[10] Brandrup, F. and Green, A. The prevalence of psoriasis in Denmark. *Acta Derm Venereol.,* 1981 61, 344-346.

[11] Gelfand, J.M., et al. Prevalence and treatment of psoriasis in the United Kingdom: a population-based study. *Arch. Dermatol,* 2005 141, 1537-1541.

[12] Henseler, T. and Christophers, E. Psoriasis of early and late onset: characterization of two types of psoriasis vulgaris. *J. Am. Acad. Dermatol*, 1985 13, 450-456.
[13] Ferrandiz, C., et al. Prevalence of psoriasis in Spain (Epiderma Project: phase I). *J. Eur Acad Dermatol. Venereol.*, 2001 15, 20-23.
[14] Canadian Psoriasis Guidelines Committee. Canadian Guidelines for the Management of Plaque Psoriasis, June 2009. http://www.dermatology.ca/psoriasisguidelines.
[15] Griffiths, C.E., et al. A classification of psoriasis vulgaris according to phenotype. *Br. J. Dermatol.,* 2007 156, 258-262.
[16] American Academy of Dermatology. Guidelines of care for the management of psoriasis and psoriatic arthritis. *J. Am. Acad. Dermatol.*, 2008 58, 826-850.
[17] Griffiths, C.E. and Barker, J.N. Pathogenesis and clinical features of psoriasis. *Lancet,* 2007 370, 263-271.
[18] Fredriksson, T. and Pettersson, U. Severe psoriasis—oral therapy with a new retinoid. *Dermatologica*, 1978 157, 238-244.
[19] Feldman, S.R. and Krueger, G.G. Psoriasis assessment tools in clinical trials. *Ann. Rheum. Dis*, 2005 64 Suppl 2, ii65-68; discussion ii69-73.
[20] Ellis, C.N. and Krueger, G.G. Treatment of chronic plaque psoriasis by selective targeting of memory effector T lymphocytes. *N. Engl. J. Med.*, 2001 345, 248-255.
[21] Mease, P.J., et al. Etanercept in the treatment of psoriatic arthritis and psoriasis: a randomized trial. *Lancet,* 2000 356, 385-390.
[22] Carlin, C.S., et al. A 50% reduction in the Psoriasis Area and Severity Index (PASI 50) is a clinically significant endpoint in the assessment of psoriasis. *J. Am. Acad. Dermatol.,* 2004 50, 859-866.
[23] Lowes, M.A.; Bowcock, A.M. and Krueger, J.G. Pathogenesis and therapy of psoriasis. *Nature*, 2007 445, 866-873.
[24] Schon, M.P. and Boehncke, W.H. Psoriasis. *N. Engl. J. Med.*, 2005 352, 1899-1912.
[25] Barker, J.N., et al. Preferential adherence of T lymphocytes and neutrophils to psoriatic epidermis. *Br. J. Dermatol.*, 1992 127, 205-211.
[26] Van de Kerkhof, P.C. and Lammers, A.M. Intraepidermal accumulation of polymorphonuclear leukocytes in chronic stable plaque psoriasis. *Dermatologica,* 1987 174, 224-227.
[27] Creamer, D., et al. Angiogenesis in psoriasis. *Angiogenesis*, 2002 5, 231-236.

[28] Heidenreich, R.; Rocken, M. and Ghoreschi, K. Angiogenesis drives psoriasis pathogenesis. *Int. J. Exp. Pathol.*, 2009 90, 232-248.
[29] Krueger, J.G and Bowcock, A. Psoriasis pathophysiology: current concepts of pathogenesis. *Ann. Rheum. Dis*, 2005 64 Suppl 2, ii30-ii36.
[30] Bowcock, A.M. The genetics of psoriasis and autoimmunity. *Annu. Rev. Genomics Hum. Genet*, 2005 6, 93-122.
[31] Sullivan-Whalen, M. and Gilleaudeau, P. Psoriasis: hope for the future. *Nurs. Clin. North Am.*, 2007 42, 467-484, vii.
[32] Hwu, W.L., et al. Mapping of psoriasis to 17q terminus. *J Med Genet*, 2005 42, 152-158.
[33] Capon, F., et al. Haplotype analysis of distantly related populations implicates corneodesmosin in psoriasis susceptibility. *J. Med. Genet*, 2003 40, 447-452.
[34] Laptev, M.V. and Nikulin, N.K. Synchronization of oscillations of proliferation of keratinocytes in psoriatic skin by external periodic force: a mathematical model. *J. Theor Biol.*, 2005 235, 485-494.
[35] Detmar, M., et al. Initial hyperproliferation and incomplete terminal differentiation of cultured human keratinocytes from lesional and uninvolved psoriatic skin. *Acta Derm. Venereol*, 1990 70, 295-299.
[36] Mils, V., et al. Comparative analysis of normal and psoriatic skin both in vivo and in vitro. *Differentiation,* 1994 58, 77-86.
[37] Paramio, J.M., et al. Modulation of cell proliferation by cytokeratins K10 and K16. *Mol. Cell Biol.,* 1999 19, 3086-3094.
[38] Santos, M., et al. The expression of keratin k10 in the basal layer of the epidermis inhibits cell proliferation and prevents skin tumorigenesis. *J. Biol. Chem*, 2002 277, 19122-19130.
[39] Bhawan, J., et al. K16 expression in uninvolved psoriatic skin: a possible marker of pre-clinical psoriasis. *J. Cutan Pathol.*, 2004 31, 471-476.
[40] Leigh, I.M., et al. Keratins (K16 and K17) as markers of keratinocyte hyperproliferation in psoriasis in vivo and in vitro. *Br. J. Dermatol,* 1995 133, 501-511.
[41] Presland, R.B., et al. Barrier function in transgenic mice overexpressing K16, involucrin, and filaggrin in the suprabasal epidermis. *J. Invest Dermatol.*, 2004 123, 603-606.
[42] Hohl, D. Expression patterns of loricrin in dermatological disorders. *Am. J. Dermatopathol.*, 1993 15, 20-27.
[43] Stoler, A., et al. Use of monospecific antisera and cRNA probes to localize the major changes in keratin expression during normal and abnormal epidermal differentiation. *J. Cell Biol.*, 1988 107, 427-446.

[44] McKay, I.A. and Leigh, I.M. Altered keratinocyte growth and differentiation in psoriasis. *Clin. Dermatol.*, 1995 13, 105-114.

[45] Schroeder, W.T., et al. Type I keratinocyte transglutaminase: expression in human skin and psoriasis. *J. Invest Dermatol.*, 1992 99, 27-34.

[46] Ishida-Yamamoto, A., et al. Immunoelectron microscopic analysis of cornified cell envelope formation in normal and psoriatic epidermis. *J. Histochem. Cytochem,* 1996 44, 167-175.

[47] Vaccaro, M., et al. Changes in the distribution of laminin alpha1 chain in psoriatic skin: immunohistochemical study using confocal laser scanning microscopy. *Br. J. Dermatol*, 2002 146, 392-398.

[48] Smetsers, T.F., et al. Human single-chain antibodies reactive with native chondroitin sulfate detect chondroitin sulfate alterations in melanoma and psoriasis. *J. Invest Dermatol.*, 2004 122, 707-716.

[49] Black, A.F., et al. Optimization and characterization of an engineered human skin equivalent. *Tissue Eng*, 2005 11, 723-733.

[50] Hynes, R.O. *Fibronectins.* Edition. New York: Springer-Verlag; 1990.

[51] Fuchs, J., et al. Redox-modulated pathways in inflammatory skin diseases. *Free Radical Biology and Medicine*, 2001 30, 337-353.

[52] Briganti, S. and Picardo, M. Antioxidant activity, lipid peroxidation and skin diseases. What's new. *Journal of the European Academy of Dermatology and Venereology*, 2003 17, 663-669.

[53] Trouba, K.J., et al. Oxidative stress and its role in skin disease. *Antioxidants and Redox Signaling,* 2002 4, 665-673.

[54] Pelle, E., et al. Keratinocytes act as a source of reactive oxygen species by transferring hydrogen peroxide to melanocytes. *Journal of Investigative Dermatology*, 2005 124, 793-797.

[55] Ginsburg, I. and Kohen, R. Cell-damage in inflammatory and infectious sites might involve a coordinated cross-talk among oxidants, microbial hemolysins and ampiphiles, cationic proteins, phospholipases, fatty-acids, proteinases and cytokines (an overview). *Free Radical Research*, 1995 22, 489-517.

[56] Lee, S.H.; Jeong, S.K. and Ahn, S.K. An update of the defensive barrier function of skin. *Yonsei Medical Journal*, 2006 47, 293-306.

[57] Motta, S., et al. Abnormality of water barrier function in psoriasis— role of ceramide fractions. *Archives of Dermatology*, 1994 130, 452-456.

[58] Elias, P.M. and Feingold, K.R. Does the tail wag the dog? Role of the barrier in the pathogenesis of inflammatory dermatoses and therapeutic implications. *Archives of Dermatology,* 2001 137, 1079-1081.

[59] Shilov, V.N. and Sergienko, V.I. Oxidative stress in keratinocytes as an etiopathogenetic factor of psoriasis. *Bull. Exp. Biol. Med.*, 2000 129, 309-313.
[60] Kural, B.V., et al. Evaluation of the atherogenic tendency of lipids and lipoprotein content and their relationships with oxidant-antioxidant system in patients with psoriasis. *Clinica Chimica Acta*, 2003 328, 71-82.
[61] Kokcam, I. and Naziroglu, M. Antioxidants and lipid peroxidation status in the blood of patients with psoriasis. *Clin. Chim. Acta*, 1999 289, 23-31.
[62] Fairris, G.M., et al. The effect of supplementation with selenium and vitamin-E in psoriasis. *Annals of Clinical Biochemistry*, 1989 26, 83-88.
[63] Rocha-Pereira, P., et al. The inflammatory response in mild and in severe psoriasis. *Br. J. Dermatol.*, 2004 150, 917-928.
[64] Therond, P., et al. Antioxidant enzymes in psoriatic fibroblasts and erythrocytes. *Journal of Investigative Dermatology*, 1996 106, 1325-1328.
[65] Rocha-Pereira, P., et al. Erythrocyte damage in mild and severe psoriasis. *British Journal of Dermatology*, 2004 150, 232-244.
[66] Drewa, G., et al. Activity of superoxide dismutase and catalase and the level of lipid peroxidation products reactive with TBA in patients with psoriasis. *Med. Sci. Monit*, 2002 8, BR338-343.
[67] Karaman, A.; Aliagaoglu, C. and Pirim, I. Sister chromatid exchange analysis in patients with psoriasis. *Experimental Dermatology*, 2008 17, 524-529.
[68] Utas, S., et al. Antioxidant potential of propylthiouracil in patients with psoriasis. *Clin. Biochem.*, 2002 35, 241-246.
[69] Yildirim, M., et al. The role of oxidants and antioxidants in psoriasis. *Journal of the European Academy of Dermatology and Venereology*, 2003 17, 34-36.
[70] Baz, K., et al. Oxidant/antioxidant status in patients with psoriasis. *Yonsei Medical Journal*, 2003 44, 987-990.
[71] Gokhale, N.R., et al. A study of serum nitric oxide levels in psoriasis. *Indian journal of dermatology, venereology and leprology*, 2005 71, 175-178.
[72] Zalewska, A., et al. Nitric oxide levels in plasma and fibroblast cultures of psoriasis vulgaris patients. *J. Dermatol. Sci.*, 2007 48, 237-240.
[73] Gornicki, A. and Gutsze, A. Erythrocyte membrane fluidity changes in psoriasis: an EPR study. *J. Dermatol Sci*, 2001 27, 27-30.

[74] Dimon-Gadal, S., et al. Increased oxidative damage to fibroblasts in skin with and without lesions in psoriasis. *Journal of Investigative Dermatology*, 2000 114, 984-989.
[75] Kizaki, H.; Matsuo, I. and Sakurada, T. Xanthine oxidase and guanase activities in normal and psoriatic epidermis. *Clin. Chim. Acta*, 1977 75, 1-4.
[76] Young, C.N., et al. Reactive oxygen species in tumor necrosis factor-alpha-activated primary human keratinocytes: implications for psoriasis and inflammatory skin disease. *J. Invest Dermatol.*, 2008 128, 2606-2614.
[77] Kobayashi, T., et al. Superoxide dismutase in psoriasis, squamous cell carcinoma and basal cell epithelioma: an immunohistochemical study. *Br. J. Dermatol*, 1991 124, 555-559.
[78] Lontz, W., et al. Increased messenger-RNA expression of manganese superoxide-dismutase in psoriasis skin-lesions and in cultured human keratinocytes exposed to IL-1 beta and TNF-alpha. *Free Radical Biology and Medicine*, 1995 18, 349-355.
[79] Midorikawa, K. and Kawanishi, S. Superoxide dismutases enhance H2O2-induced DNA damage and alter its site specificity. *Febs Letters*, 2001 495, 187-190.
[80] Ormerod, A.D., et al. Detection of nitric oxide and nitric oxide synthases in psoriasis. *Arch. Dermatol Res.*, 1998 290, 3-8.
[81] Leveque, N., et al. In vivo assessment of iron and ascorbic acid in psoriatic dermis. Acta *Derm. Venereol.*, 2004 84, 2-5.
[82] Pujari V., SA, Ireddy S. Oxidant and antioxidant status in psoriatic patients. *Biomedical research*, 2010 21, 221-223.
[83] Relhan, V., et al. Blood thiols and malondialdehyde levels in psoriasis. *J. Dermatol.*, 2002 29, 399-403.
[84] Gerbaud, P., et al. Differential regulation of Cu, Zn- and Mn-superoxide dismutases by retinoic acid in normal and psoriatic human fibroblasts. *Journal of Autoimmunity*, 2005 24, 69-78.
[85] Majewski, S., et al. Decreased levels of vitamin A in serum of patients with psoriasis. *Arch. Dermatol. Res.*, 1989 280, 499-501.
[86] Sabat, R., et al. Immunopathogenesis of psoriasis. *Exp. Dermatol.*, 2007 16, 779-798.
[87] Bowcock, A.M. and Krueger, J.G. Getting under the skin: the immunogenetics of psoriasis. *Nat. Re. Immunol.*, 2005 5, 699-711.
[88] Nestle, F.O.; Kaplan, D.H. and Barker, J. Psoriasis. *N Engl. J. Med.*, 2009 361, 496-509.

[89] Lew, W.; Bowcock, A.M. and Krueger, J.G. Psoriasis vulgaris: cutaneous lymphoid tissue supports T-cell activation and "Type 1" inflammatory gene expression. *Trends Immunol*, 2004 25, 295-305.

[90] Giustizieri, M.L., et al. Keratinocytes from patients with atopic dermatitis and psoriasis show a distinct chemokine production profile in response to T cell-derived cytokines. *J Allergy Clin. Immunol.*, 2001 107, 871-877.

[91] Albanesi, C.; Cavani, A. and Girolomoni, G. Interferon-gamma-stimulated human keratinocytes express the genes necessary for the production of peptide-loaded MHC class II molecules. *J. Invest Dermatol.*, 1998 110, 138-142.

[92] Dustin, M.L., et al. Adhesion of T lymphoblasts to epidermal keratinocytes is regulated by interferon gamma and is mediated by intercellular adhesion molecule 1 (ICAM-1). *J. Exp. Med.*, 1988 167, 1323-1340.

[93] Di Cesare, A.; Di Meglio, P. and Nestle, F.O. The IL-23/Th17 axis in the immunopathogenesis of psoriasis. *J. Invest Dermatol.*, 2009 129, 1339-1350.

[94] Lowes, M.A., et al. Psoriasis vulgaris lesions contain discrete populations of Th1 and Th17 T cells. *J. Invest Dermatol.*, 2008 128, 1207-1211.

[95] Bettelli, E.; Oukka, M. and Kuchroo, V.K. T(H)-17 cells in the circle of immunity and autoimmunity. *Nat. Immunol*, 2007 8, 345-350.

[96] Nograles, K.E., et al. Th17 cytokines interleukin (IL)-17 and IL-22 modulate distinct inflammatory and keratinocyte-response pathways. *Br. J. Dermatol*, 2008 159, 1092-1102.

[97] Griffiths, C.E., et al. Comparison of ustekinumab and etanercept for moderate-to-severe psoriasis. *N Engl. J. Med.*, 2010 362, 118-128.

[98] Eyerich, S., et al. Th22 cells represent a distinct human T cell subset involved in epidermal immunity and remodeling. *J. Clin. Invest*, 2009 119, 3573-3585.

[99] Kagami, S., et al. Circulating Th17, Th22, and Th1 cells are increased in psoriasis. *J. Invest Dermatol.*, 2010 130, 1373-1383.

[100] Balato, A.; Unutmaz, D. and Gaspari, A.A. Natural killer T cells: an unconventional T-cell subset with diverse effector and regulatory functions. *J. Invest Dermatol.*, 2009 129, 1628-1642.

[101] Peternel, S. and Kastelan, M. Immunopathogenesis of psoriasis: focus on natural killer T cells. *J. Eur. Acad. Dermatol. Venereol.*, 2009 23, 1123-1127.

[102] Gilhar, A., et al. Psoriasis is mediated by a cutaneous defect triggered by activated immunocytes: induction of psoriasis by cells with natural killer receptors. *J. Invest Dermatol.*, 2002 119, 384-391.

[103] Vissers, W.H., et al. The effect of the combination of calcipotriol and betamethasone dipropionate versus both monotherapies on epidermal proliferation, keratinization and T-cell subsets in chronic plaque psoriasis. *Exp. Dermatol.*, 2004 13, 106-112.

[104] Bovenschen, H.J., et al. Explorative immunohistochemical study to evaluate the addition of a topical corticosteroid in the early phase of alefacept treatment for psoriasis. *Arch. Dermatol. Res.*, 2007 298, 457-463.

[105] Nestle, F.O., et al. Skin immune sentinels in health and disease. *Nat. Rev. Immunol.*, 2009 9, 679-691.

[106] Nickoloff, B.J.; Qin, J.Z. and Nestle, F.O. Immunopathogenesis of psoriasis. *Clin. Rev. Allergy Immunol.*, 2007 33, 45-56.

[107] Jariwala, S.P. The role of dendritic cells in the immunopathogenesis of psoriasis. *Arch. Dermatol. Res.*, 2007 299, 359-366.

[108] Chamian, F. and Krueger, J.G. Psoriasis vulgaris: interplay of T lymphocytes, dendritic cells, and inflammatory cytokines in pathogenesis. *Curr. Opin. Rheumatol.*, 2004 16, 331-337.

[109] Terui, T.; Ozawa, M. and Tagami, H. Role of neutrophils in induction of acute inflammation in T-cell-mediated immune dermatosis, psoriasis: a neutrophil-associated inflammation-boosting loop. *Exp. Dermatol.*, 2000 9, 1-10.

[110] Toichi, E.; Tachibana, T. and Furukawa, F. Rapid improvement of psoriasis vulgaris during drug-induced agranulocytosis. *J. Am. Acad. Dermatol.*, 2000 43, 391-395.

[111] Rahmoun, M., et al. Cytokine-induced CEACAM1 expression on keratinocytes is characteristic for psoriatic skin and contributes to a prolonged lifespan of neutrophils. *J. Invest Dermatol.*, 2009 129, 671-681.

[112] Keller, M., et al. T cell-regulated neutrophilic inflammation in autoinflammatory diseases. *J. Immunol.*, 2005 175, 7678-7686.

[113] Schaerli, P., et al. Characterization of human T cells that regulate neutrophilic skin inflammation. *J. Immunol.*, 2004 173, 2151-2158.

[114] Seifert, O.; Holmberg, J. and Linnarsson, B.M. Decreased activity of neutrophil glutathione peroxidase in chronic plaque-type psoriasis. *J. Am. Acad. Dermatol.*, 2007 57, 528-529.

[115] Harvima, I.T., et al. Is there a role for mast cells in psoriasis? *Arch. Dermatol Res.*, 2008 300, 461-478.
[116] Jiang, W.Y., et al. Mast cell density and IL-8 expression in nonlesional and lesional psoriatic skin. *Int. J. Dermatol.*, 2001 40, 699-703.
[117] Mekori, Y.A. and Metcalfe, D.D. Mast cell-T cell interactions. *J. Allergy Clin. Immunol.*, 1999 104, 517-523.
[118] Kunz, M. and Ibrahim, S.M. Cytokines and cytokine profiles in human autoimmune diseases and animal models of autoimmunity. *Mediators Inflamm*, 2009, 979258.
[119] Nickoloff, B.J., et al. The cytokine and chemokine network in psoriasis. *Clin. Dermatol.*, 2007 25, 568-573.
[120] Nickoloff, B.J. Cracking the cytokine code in psoriasis. *Nat. Med.*, 2007 13, 242-244.
[121] Tonel, G. and Conrad, C. Interplay between keratinocytes and immune cells—recent insights into psoriasis pathogenesis. *Int. J. Biochem. Cell Biol.*, 2009 41, 963-968.
[122] Farber, E.M. and Nall, M.L. The natural history of psoriasis in 5,600 patients. *Dermatologica*, 1974 148, 1-18.
[123] Elder, J.T. Genome-wide association scan yields new insights into the immunopathogenesis of psoriasis. *Genes Immun*, 2009 10, 201-209.
[124] Fan, X., et al. Fine mapping of the psoriasis susceptibility locus PSORS1 supports HLA-C as the susceptibility gene in the Han Chinese population. *PLoS Genet*, 2008 4, e1000038.
[125] Elder, J.T. PSORS1: linking genetics and immunology. *J. Invest. Dermatol.*, 2006 126, 1205-1206.
[126] Nair, R.P., et al. Sequence and haplotype analysis supports HLA-C as the psoriasis susceptibility 1 gene. *Am. J. Hum. Genet.*, 2006 78, 827-851.
[127] Stuart, P.E., et al. Comparison of MHC class I risk haplotypes in Thai and Caucasian psoriatics shows locus heterogeneity at PSORS1. *Tissue Antigens*, 2010
[128] Tomfohrde, J., et al. Gene for familial psoriasis susceptibility mapped to the distal end of human chromosome 17q. *Science*, 1994 264, 1141-1145.
[129] Duffin, K.C. and Krueger, G.G. Genetic variations in cytokines and cytokine receptors associated with psoriasis found by genome-wide association. *J. Invest. Dermatol.*, 2009 129, 827-833.

[130] Asumalahti, K., et al. Genetic analysis of PSORS1 distinguishes guttate psoriasis and palmoplantar pustulosis. *J. Invest Dermatol.*, 2003 120, 627-632.
[131] Allen, M.H., et al. The major psoriasis susceptibility locus PSORS1 is not a risk factor for late-onset psoriasis. *J. Invest. Dermatol.*, 2005 124, 103-106.
[132] Helms, C., et al. A putative RUNX1 binding site variant between SLC9A3R1 and NAT9 is associated with susceptibility to psoriasis. *Nat. Genet*, 2003 35, 349-356.
[133] Morar, N., et al. Investigation of the chromosome 17q25 PSORS2 locus in atopic dermatitis. *J. Invest Dermatol.*, 2006 126, 603-606.
[134] Huffmeier, U., et al. Lack of evidence for genetic association to RUNX1 binding site at PSORS2 in different German psoriasis cohorts. *J. Invest Dermatol.*, 2005 124, 107-110.
[135] Stuart, P., et al. Analysis of RUNX1 binding site and RAPTOR polymorphisms in psoriasis: no evidence for association despite adequate power and evidence for linkage. *J. Med. Genet.*, 2006 43, 12-17.
[136] Capon, F., et al. Fine mapping of the PSORS4 psoriasis susceptibility region on chromosome 1q21. *J. Invest Dermatol.*, 2001 116, 728-730.
[137] de Cid, R., et al. Deletion of the late cornified envelope LCE3B and LCE3C genes as a susceptibility factor for psoriasis. *Nat. Genet*, 2009 41, 211-215.
[138] Liu, Y., et al. A genome-wide association study of psoriasis and psoriatic arthritis identifies new disease loci. *PLoS Genet*, 2008 4, e1000041.
[139] Huffmeier, U., et al. Replication of LCE3C-LCE3B CNV as a risk factor for psoriasis and analysis of interaction with other genetic risk factors. *J. Invest Dermatol.*, 2010 130, 979-984.
[140] Zhang, X.J., et al. Psoriasis genome-wide association study identifies susceptibility variants within LCE gene cluster at 1q21. *Nat Genet*, 2009 41, 205-210.
[141] Bergboer, J.G., et al. Deletion of Late Cornified Envelope 3B and 3C genes is not associated with atopic dermatitis. *J. Invest Dermatol.*, 2010 130, 2057-2061.
[142] Nair, R.P., et al. Genome-wide scan reveals association of psoriasis with IL-23 and NF-kappaB pathways. *Nat. Genet*, 2009 41, 199-204.
[143] Elder, J.T., et al. Molecular dissection of psoriasis: integrating genetics and biology. *J. Invest Dermatol*, 2010 130, 1213-1226.

[144] Cargill, M., et al. A large-scale genetic association study confirms IL12B and leads to the identification of IL23R as psoriasis-risk genes. *Am. J. Hum. Genet*, 2007 80, 273-290.

[145] Filer, C.E., et al. Investigation of association of genes NAT9, SLC9A3R1 and RAPTOR on chromosome 17q25 with psoriatic arthritis. *Ann. Rheum. Dis.*, 2009 68, 292-293.

[146] Tsunemi, Y., et al. Interleukin-12 p40 gene (IL12B) 3'-untranslated region polymorphism is associated with susceptibility to atopic dermatitis and psoriasis vulgaris. *J. Dermatol. Sci.*, 2002 30, 161-166.

[147] Capon, F., et al. Sequence variants in the genes for the interleukin-23 receptor (IL23R) and its ligand (IL12B) confer protection against psoriasis. *Hum. Genet*, 2007 122, 201-206.

[148] Nair, R.P., et al. Polymorphisms of the IL12B and IL23R genes are associated with psoriasis. *J. Invest Dermatol.*, 2008 128, 1653-1661.

[149] Segal, B.M., et al. Repeated subcutaneous injections of IL12/23 p40 neutralizing antibody, ustekinumab, in patients with relapsing-remitting multiple sclerosis: a phase II, double-blind, placebo-controlled, randomized, dose-ranging study. *Lancet Neurol*, 2008 7, 796-804.

[150] Duerr, R.H., et al. A genome-wide association study identifies IL23R as an inflammatory bowel disease gene. *Science,* 2006 314, 1461-1463.

[151] Duffin, K.C.; Woodcock, J. and Krueger, G.G. Genetic variations associated with psoriasis and psoriatic arthritis found by genome-wide association. *Dermatol. Ther.*, 2010 23, 101-113.

[152] Chang, M., et al. Variants in the 5q31 cytokine gene cluster are associated with psoriasis. *Genes Immun*, 2008 9, 176-181.

[153] Newcomb, D.C., et al. A functional IL-13 receptor is expressed on polarized murine CD4+ Th17 cells and IL-13 signaling attenuates Th17 cytokine production. *J. Immunol*, 2009 182, 5317-5321.

[154] Li, Y., et al. The 5q31 variants associated with psoriasis and Crohn's disease are distinct. *Hum. Mol. Genet*, 2008 17, 2978-2985.

[155] Vang, T., et al. Protein tyrosine phosphatase PTPN22 in human autoimmunity. *Autoimmunity*, 2007 40, 453-461.

[156] Li, Y., et al. Further genetic evidence for three psoriasis-risk genes: ADAM33, CDKAL1, and PTPN22. *J. Invest Dermatol.*, 2009 129, 629-634.

[157] Huffmeier, U., et al. Evidence for susceptibility determinant(s) to psoriasis vulgaris in or near PTPN22 in German patients. *J. Med. Genet*, 2006 43, 517-522.

[158] Smith, R.L., et al. Polymorphisms in the PTPN22 region are associated with psoriasis of early onset. *Br. J. Dermatol*, 2008 158, 962-968.
[159] Capon, F., et al. Identification of ZNF313/RNF114 as a novel psoriasis susceptibility gene. *Hum. Mol. Genet.*, 2008 17, 1938-1945.
[160] Liu, Y.C.; Penninger, J. and Karin, M. Immunity by ubiquitylation: a reversible process of modification. *Nat Rev. Immunol.*, 2005 5, 941-952.
[161] Vinuesa, C.G., et al. A RING-type ubiquitin ligase family member required to repress follicular helper T cells and autoimmunity. *Nature*, 2005 435, 452-458.
[162] Quaranta, M., et al. Differential contribution of CDKAL1 variants to psoriasis, Crohn's disease and type II diabetes. *Genes Immun*, 2009 10, 654-658.
[163] Wolf, N., et al. Psoriasis is associated with pleiotropic susceptibility loci identified in type II diabetes and Crohn's disease. *J. Med. Genet*, 2008 45, 114-116.
[164] Mease, P.J. and Menter, M.A. Quality-of-life issues in psoriasis and psoriatic arthritis: outcome measures and therapies from a dermatological perspective. *J. Am. Acad. Dermatol.*, 2006 54, 685-704.
[165] Fitzpatrick, T.B. and Wolff, K. *Fitzpatrick's dermatology in general medicine*. Seventh edition. New York: Medical, M-H; 2008.
[166] Bagel, J. Topical therapies for the treatment of plaque psoriasis. *Cutis*, 2009 84, 3-13.
[167] Fadzil, M.H., et al. Area assessment of psoriasis lesions for PASI scoring. *J. Med. Eng. Technol*, 2009 33, 426-436.
[168] Bessis, D., et al. Le psoriasis en médecine générale. Edition. *Rueil-Malmaison: Arnette*; 2005.
[169] Camisa, C. *Handbook of psoriasis*. Second edition. Oxford: Publishing, B; 2004.
[170] Thielen, A.M. and Laffitte, E. [Topical treatments for psoriasis in 2009]. *Rev. Med. Suisse*, 2009 5, 876, 878-881.
[171] Del Rosso, J. and Friedlander, S.F. Corticosteroids: options in the era of steroid-sparing therapy. *J. Am. Acad. Dermatol.*, 2005 53, S50-58.
[172] Raymond, G.P. and Houle, M-C. Présentation des corticostéroïdes pour le traitement du psoriasis. *Skin Pharmacies*, 2007 2,
[173] Kamili, Q.U. and Menter, A. Topical treatment of psoriasis. *Curr. Probl Dermatol.*, 2009 38, 37-58.
[174] Norris, D.A. Mechanisms of action of topical therapies and the rationale for combination therapy. *J. Am. Acad. Dermatol.*, 2005 53, S17-25.

[175] Lebwohl, M. The role of salicylic acid in the treatment of psoriasis. *Int. J. Dermatol*, 1999 38, 16-24.

[176] Tanghetti, E.A. The role of topical vitamin D modulators in psoriasis therapy. *J. Drugs* Dermatol, 2009 8 Suppl 8, 4-8.

[177] Gold, L.F. Calcitriol ointment: optimizing psoriasis therapy. *J. Drugs Dermatol.*, 2009 8 Suppl 8, 23-27.

[178] Tremblay, J-F., R. Bissonnette. Topical Agent for the Treatment of Psoriasis, Past, Present and Future. *J. Cutan Med. Surg.*, 2002 10, 8-11.

[179] Attar, M., et al. Disposition and biotransformation of the acetylenic retinoid tazarotene in humans. *J. Pharm. Sci*, 2005 94, 2246-2255.

[180] Lebwohl, M.; Ting, P.T. and Koo, J.Y. Psoriasis treatment: traditional therapy. *Ann. Rheum. Dis.*, 2005 64 Suppl 2, ii83-86.

[181] Lemay, R. Pharmacothérapie du psoriasis. *Québec Pharmacie*, 2006 53, 141-150.

[182] Paghdal, K.V. and Schwartz, R.A. Topical tar: back to the future. *J. Am. Acad. Dermatol.*, 2009 61, 294-302.

[183] Nicolas, J-F. and Thivolet, J. Psoriasis: de la clinique à la thérapeutique. Edition. Paris: Eurotext, JL; 1997.

[184] Grundmann-Kollmann, M., et al. Narrowband UVB and cream psoralen-UVA combination therapy for plaque-type psoriasis. *J. Am. Acad. Dermatol.*, 2004 50, 734-739.

[185] Grundmann, S.A. and Beissert, S. Regulation of cellular immunity by Photo(chemo)therapy. *Front Biosci*, 2009 14, 4326-4336.

[186] Nguyen, T., et al. Practice of phototherapy in the treatment of moderate-to-severe psoriasis. *Curr. Probl Dermatol*, 2009 38, 59-78.

[187] Lee, M. and Kalb, R.E. Systemic therapy for psoriasis. *Dermatol Nurs*, 2008 20, 105-111; quiz 112.

[188] Ghoreschi, K.; Mrowietz, U. and Rocken, M. A molecule solves psoriasis? Systemic therapies for psoriasis inducing interleukin 4 and Th2 responses. *J. Mol. Med.*, 2003 81, 471-480.

[189] Zakarian, K., et al. Excimer laser for psoriasis: a review of theories regarding enhanced efficacy over traditional UVB phototherapy. *J. Drugs Dermatol.*, 2007 6, 794-798.

[190] Dubertret, L. Le psoriasis: de la clinique à la thérapeutique. Edition. *MED'COM*; 2004.

[191] Deng, H., et al. Photochemotherapy inhibits angiogenesis and induces apoptosis of endothelial cells in vitro. *Photodermatol Photoimmunol Photomed*, 2004 20, 191-199.

[192] Dubertret, L. Retinoids, methotrexate and cyclosporine. *Curr. Probl Dermatol*, 2009 38, 79-94.
[193] Heenen, M., et al. Methotrexate induces apoptotic cell death in human keratinocytes. *Arch. Dermatol. Res.*, 1998 290, 240-245.
[194] Johnston, A., et al. The anti-inflammatory action of methotrexate is not mediated by lymphocyte apoptosis, but by the suppression of activation and adhesion molecules. *Clin. Immunol.*, 2005 114, 154-163.
[195] Carlin, C.S.; Callis, K.P. and Krueger, G.G. Efficacy of acitretin and commercial tanning bed therapy for psoriasis. *Arch. Dermatol.*, 2003 139, 436-442.
[196] Pang, M.L.; Murase, J.E. and Koo, J. An updated review of acitretin—a systemic retinoid for the treatment of psoriasis. *Expert Opin. Drug Metab. Toxicol*, 2008 4, 953-964.
[197] Karashima, T.; Hachisuka, H. and Sasai, Y. FK506 and cyclosporin A inhibit growth factor-stimulated human keratinocyte proliferation by blocking cells in the G0/G1 phases of the cell cycle. *J. Dermatol Sci.*, 1996 12, 246-254.
[198] Weinberg, J.M. An overview of infliximab, etanercept, efalizumab, and alefacept as biologic therapy for psoriasis. *Clin. Ther*, 2003 25, 2487-2505.
[199] Singri, P.; West, D.P. and Gordon, K.B. Biologic therapy for psoriasis: the new therapeutic frontier. *Arch. Dermatol.*, 2002 138, 657-663.
[200] Tzu, J., et al. Biological agents in the treatment of psoriasis. *G Ital. Dermatol. Venereol.*, 2008 143, 315-327.
[201] Kormeili, T.; Lowe, N.J. and Yamauchi, P.S. Psoriasis: immunopathogenesis and evolving immunomodulators and systemic therapies; U.S. experiences. *Br. J. Dermatol.*, 2004 151, 3-15.
[202] Thielen, A.M. and Marazza, G. [The biological treatments for moderate to severe plaque psoriasis]. *Rev. Med. Suisse*, 2008 4, 1089-1090, 1092-1084.
[203] Altomare, G., et al. Etanercept provides a more physiological approach in the treatment of psoriasis. *Dermatol. Ther.*, 2008 21 Suppl 2, S1-14.
[204] Papoutsaki, M., et al. Adalimumab for the treatment of severe psoriasis and psoriatic arthritis. *Expert Opin. Biol. Ther.*, 2008 8, 363-370.
[205] Papp, K.A. Monitoring biologics for the treatment of psoriasis. *Clin. Dermatol.*, 2008 26, 515-521.
[206] Heffernan, M.P. and Leonardi, C.L. Alefacept for psoriasis. *Semin. Cutan Med. Surg.*, 2010 29, 53-55.

[207] Lev-Tov, H. and Hadi, S. Alefacept—a drug review. *Rev. Recent Clin Trials*, 2006 1, 163-164.
[208] Papp, K.A. Monitoring patients treated with efalizumab or alefacept. *Curr. Probl. Dermatol.*, 2009 38, 95-106.
[209] Lima, X.T., et al. Briakinumab. *Expert Opin. Biol. Ther.*, 2009 9, 1107-1113.
[210] Gudjonsson, J.E., et al. Mouse models of psoriasis. *J. Invest. Dermatol.*, 2007 127, 1292-1308.
[211] Tjabringa, G., et al. Development and validation of human psoriatic skin equivalents. *Am. J. Pathol.*, 2008 173, 815-823.
[212] Sundberg, J.P., et al. Inherited mouse mutations as models of human adnexal, cornification, and papulosquamous dermatoses. *J. Invest. Dermatol.*, 1990 95, 62S-63S.
[213] Mizutani, H., et al. Animal models of psoriasis and pustular psoriasis. *Arch. Dermatol. Res*, 2003 295 Suppl 1, S67-68.
[214] Schon, M.P. Animal models of psoriasis: a critical appraisal. *Exp. Dermatol.*, 2008 17, 703-712.
[215] Zheng, Y., et al. Scd1 is expressed in sebaceous glands and is disrupted in the asebia mouse. *Nat. Genet.*, 1999 23, 268-270.
[216] Schon, M.P. Animal models of psoriasis - what can we learn from them? *J. Invest. Dermatol.*, 1999 112, 405-410.
[217] Jean, J. and Pouliot, R. Tissue engineering: In vivo and in vitro models of psoriasis. In: Eberli, D., editor. 2010; 359-382. http://www.intechopen.com/articles/show/title/in-vivo-and-in-vitro-models-of-psoriasis.
[218] Krueger, G.G.; Chambers, D.A. and Shelby, J. Involved and uninvolved skin from psoriatic subjects: are they equally diseased? Assessment by skin transplanted to congenitally athymic (nude) mice. *J. Clin. Invest.*, 1981 68, 1548-1557.
[219] Fraki, J.E.; Briggaman, R.A. and Lazarus, G.S. Transplantation of psoriatic skin onto nude mice. *J. Invest. Dermatol.*, 1983 80 Suppl, 31s-35s.
[220] Raychaudhuri, S.P., et al. Severe combined immunodeficiency mouse-human skin chimeras: a unique animal model for the study of psoriasis and cutaneous inflammation. *Br. J. Dermatol.*, 2001 144, 931-939.
[221] Boyman, O., et al. Spontaneous development of psoriasis in a new animal model shows an essential role for resident T cells and tumor necrosis factor-alpha. *J. Exp. Med.*, 2004 199, 731-736.

[222] Bullard, D.C., et al. A polygenic mouse model of psoriasiform skin disease in CD18-deficient mice. *Proc. Natl. Acad. Sci. USA*, 1996 93, 2116-2121.

[223] Danilenko, D.M. Review paper: preclinical models of psoriasis. *Vet. Pathol.*, 2008 45, 563-575.

[224] Keith, J.C., Jr., et al. A monoclonal antibody against kininogen reduces inflammation in the HLA-B27 transgenic rat. *Arthritis Res. Ther.*, 2005 7, R769-776.

[225] Breban, M., et al. T cells, but not thymic exposure to HLA-B27, are required for the inflammatory disease of HLA-B27 transgenic rats. *J. Immunol.*, 1996 156, 794-803.

[226] Kess, D., et al. CD4+ T cell-associated pathophysiology critically depends on CD18 gene dose effects in a murine model of psoriasis. *J. Immunol.*, 2003 171, 5697-5706.

[227] Schon, M.P., et al. Cutaneous inflammatory disorder in integrin alphaE (CD103)-deficient mice. *J. Immunol.*, 2000 165, 6583-6589.

[228] Kopp, T., et al. Inflammatory skin disease in K14/p40 transgenic mice: evidence for interleukin-12-like activities of p40. *J. Invest. Dermatol.*, 2001 117, 618-626.

[229] Voskas, D., et al. A cyclosporine-sensitive psoriasis-like disease produced in Tie2 transgenic mice. *Am. J. Pathol.*, 2005 166, 843-855.

[230] Xia, Y.P., et al. Transgenic delivery of VEGF to mouse skin leads to an inflammatory condition resembling human psoriasis. *Blood*, 2003 102, 161-168.

[231] Sano, S., et al. Stat3 links activated keratinocytes and immunocytes required for development of psoriasis in a novel transgenic mouse model. *Nat. Med.*, 2005 11, 43-49.

[232] Pasparakis, M., et al. TNF-mediated inflammatory skin disease in mice with epidermis-specific deletion of IKK2. *Nature*, 2002 417, 861-866.

[233] Zenz, R., et al. Psoriasis-like skin disease and arthritis caused by inducible epidermal deletion of Jun proteins. *Nature*, 2005 437, 369-375.

[234] Guo, L.; Yu, Q.C. and Fuchs, E. Targeting expression of keratinocyte growth factor to keratinocytes elicits striking changes in epithelial differentiation in transgenic mice. *Embo. J.*, 1993 12, 973-986.

[235] Vassar, R. and Fuchs, E. Transgenic mice provide new insights into the role of TGF-alpha during epidermal development and differentiation. *Genes. Dev.*, 1991 5, 714-727.

[236] Blumberg, H., et al. Interleukin 20: discovery, receptor identification, and role in epidermal function. *Cell*, 2001 104, 9-19.

[237] Cook, P.W., et al. Transgenic expression of the human amphiregulin gene induces a psoriasis-like phenotype. *J. Clin. Invest.*, 1997 100, 2286-2294.
[238] Groves, R.W., et al. Inflammatory skin disease in transgenic mice that express high levels of interleukin 1 alpha in basal epidermis. *Proc. Natl. Acad. Sci. USA*, 1995 92, 11874-11878.
[239] Turksen, K., et al. Interleukin 6: insights to its function in skin by overexpression in transgenic mice. *Proc. Natl. Acad. Sci. USA*, 1992 89, 5068-5072.
[240] Blessing, M.; Schirmacher, P. and Kaiser, S. Overexpression of bone morphogenetic protein-6 (BMP-6) in the epidermis of transgenic mice: inhibition or stimulation of proliferation depending on the pattern of transgene expression and formation of psoriatic lesions. *J. Cell Biol.*, 1996 135, 227-239.
[241] Carroll, J.M.; Romero, M.R. and Watt, F.M. Suprabasal integrin expression in the epidermis of transgenic mice results in developmental defects and a phenotype resembling psoriasis. *Cell*, 1995 83, 957-968.
[242] Hobbs, R.M., et al. Expression of activated MEK1 in differentiating epidermal cells is sufficient to generate hyperproliferative and inflammatory skin lesions. *J. Invest. Dermatol.*, 2004 123, 503-515.
[243] Cook, P.W., et al. Suprabasal expression of human amphiregulin in the epidermis of transgenic mice induces a severe, early-onset, psoriasis-like skin pathology: expression of amphiregulin in the basal epidermis is also associated with synovitis. *Exp. Dermatol.*, 2004 13, 347-356.
[244] Carroll, J.M., et al. Transgenic mice expressing IFN-gamma in the epidermis have eczema, hair hypopigmentation, and hair loss. *J. Invest. Dermatol.*, 1997 108, 412-422.
[245] Hansson, L., et al. Epidermal overexpression of stratum corneum chymotryptic enzyme in mice: a model for chronic itchy dermatitis. *J. Invest. Dermatol.*, 2002 118, 444-449.
[246] Saiag, P., et al. Psoriatic fibroblasts induce hyperproliferation of normal keratinocytes in a skin equivalent model in vitro. *Science*, 1985 230, 669-672.
[247] Konstantinova, N.V., et al. Interleukin-8 is induced in skin equivalents and is highest in those derived from psoriatic fibroblasts. *J. Invest. Dermatol.*, 1996 107, 615-621.
[248] Barker, C.L., et al. The development and characterization of an in vitro model of psoriasis. *J. Invest. Dermatol.*, 2004 123, 892-901.

[249] Bell, E., et al. Living tissue formed in vitro and accepted as skin-equivalent tissue of full thickness. *Science*, 1981 211, 1052-1054.
[250] Bell, E., et al. Development and use of a living skin equivalent. *Plast Reconstr Surg*, 1981 67, 386-392.
[251] Bell, E.; Ivarsson, B. and Merrill, C. Production of a tissue-like structure by contraction of collagen lattices by human fibroblasts of different proliferative potential in vitro. *Proc. Natl. Acad. Sci. USA*, 1979 76, 1274-1278.
[252] Germain, L. and Auger, F.A. Encyclopedic handbook of biomaterials and bioengineering Part B: Applications: Tissue engineered biomaterials: biological and mechanical characteristics. In: Wise, D.L., et al., editor. New York: 1995; 699-734.
[253] Auger, F.A., et al. Tissue-engineered human skin substitutes developed from collagen-populated hydrated gels: clinical and fundamental applications. *Med. Biol. Eng. Comput.*, 1998 36, 801-812.
[254] Michel, M., et al. Characterization of a new tissue-engineered human skin equivalent with hair. *In Vitro Cell Dev. Biol. Anim.*, 1999 35, 318-326.
[255] Pouliot, R., et al. Reconstructed human skin produced in vitro and grafted on athymic mice. *Transplantation*, 2002 73, 1751-1757.
[256] Jean, J., et al. Development of an in vitro psoriatic skin model by tissue engineering. *J. Dermatol. Sci.*, 2009 53, 19-25.
[257] Bernard, G., et al. Physical characterization of the stratum corneum of an in vitro psoriatic skin model by ATR-FTIR and Raman spectroscopies. *Biochim. Biophys Acta*, 2007 1770, 1317-1323.
[258] Guttman-Yassky, E. and Krueger, J.G. Psoriasis: evolution of pathogenic concepts and new therapies through phases of translational research. *Br. J. Dermatol.*, 2007 157, 1103-1115.
[259] de Mare, S., et al. Markers for proliferation and keratinization in the margin of the active psoriatic lesion. *Br. J. Dermatol.*, 1990 122, 469-475.
[260] Braverman, I.M. and Fonferko, E. Studies in cutaneous aging: II. The microvasculature. *J. Invest. Dermatol.*, 1982 78, 444-448.
[261] Mansbridge, J.N. and Knapp, A.M. The binding of Helix pomatia and Ulex europeus agglutinins to normal and psoriatic skin. *J. Invest. Dermatol.*, 1984 82, 170-175.
[262] Honigsmann, H. Phototherapy for psoriasis. *Clin Exp Dermatol*, 2001 26, 343-350.

[263] Gubner, R. Effect of aminopterin on epithelial tissues. *AMA Arch. Derm. Syphilol.*, 1951 64.
[264] Stewart, W.D.; Wallace, S.M. and Runikis, J.O. Absorption and local action of methotrexate in human and mouse skin. *Arch. Dermatol.*, 1972 106, 357-361.
[265] Weinstein, G.D.; McCullough, J.L. and Ross, P. Cell proliferation in normal epidermis. *J. Invest. Dermatol.*, 1984 82, 623-628.
[266] Mansbridge, J.N. and Knapp, A.M. Changes in keratinocyte maturation during wound healing. *J. Invest. Dermatol.*, 1987 89, 253-263.
[267] Braverman, I.M. and Sibley, J. Role of the microcirculation in the treatment and pathogenesis of psoriasis. *J. Invest. Dermatol.*, 1982 78, 12-17.
[268] Bos, J.D., et al. Immunocompetent cells in psoriasis. In situ immunophenotyping by monoclonal antibodies. *Arch. Dermatol. Res*, 1983 275, 181-189.
[269] Krueger, J.G. The immunologic basis for the treatment of psoriasis with new biologic agents. *J. Am. Acad. Dermatol.*, 2002 46, 1-23; quiz 23-26.
[270] Nickoloff, B.J., et al. Modulation of keratinocyte motility. Correlation with production of extracellular matrix molecules in response to growth promoting and antiproliferative factors. *Am. J. Pathol.*, 1988 132, 543-551.
[271] Baker, B.S., et al. The effects of cyclosporin A on T lymphocyte and dendritic cell sub-populations in psoriasis. *Br. J. Dermatol.*, 1987 116, 503-510.
[272] Wrone-Smith, T. and Nickoloff, B.J. Dermal injection of immunocytes induces psoriasis. *J. Clin. Invest.*, 1996 98, 1878-1887.
[273] Gottlieb, S.L., et al. Response of psoriasis to a lymphocyte-selective toxin (DAB389IL-2) suggests a primary immune, but not keratinocyte, pathogenic basis. *Nat. Med.*, 1995 1, 442-447.
[274] Abrams, J.R., et al. Blockade of T lymphocyte costimulation with cytotoxic T lymphocyte-associated antigen 4-immunoglobulin (CTLA4Ig) reverses the cellular pathology of psoriatic plaques, including the activation of keratinocytes, dendritic cells, and endothelial cells. *J. Exp. Med.*, 2000 192, 681-694.
[275] Abrams, J.R., et al. CTLA4Ig-mediated blockade of T-cell co-stimulation in patients with psoriasis vulgaris. *J. Clin. Invest.*, 1999 103, 1243-1252.
[276] Gottlieb, A.B. Psoriasis: emerging therapeutic strategies. *Nat. Rev. Drug Discov.*, 2005 4, 19-34.

[277] Gottlieb, A.B., et al. Infliximab monotherapy provides rapid and sustained benefit for plaque-type psoriasis. *J. Am. Acad. Dermatol.*, 2003 48, 829-835.

[278] Gugasyan, R., et al. The transcription factors c-rel and RelA control epidermal development and homeostasis in embryonic and adult skin via distinct mechanisms. *Mol. Cell Biol.*, 2004 24, 5733-5745.

[279] Gottlieb, A.B., et al. Pharmacodynamic and pharmacokinetic response to anti-tumor necrosis factor-alpha monoclonal antibody (infliximab) treatment of moderate to severe psoriasis vulgaris. *J. Am. Acad. Dermatol.*, 2003 48, 68-75.

Index

A

Acitretin, 23, 29
Adalimumab, 23, 30, 58
Adhesion, 10, 16, 28, 58
Adverse effects, 30
Age, 2, 18
Agranulocytosis, 16, 52
Alefacept, 23, 31, 58
Allergic reaction, 16
Anaphylactic shock, 30
Angiogenesis, 4, 5, 11, 16, 46, 47, 57
Antibody, 20, 30, 31, 55
Antigen, 9, 15, 27, 31, 41, 63
Antigen-presenting cell, 41
Antioxidant, 9, 10, 49, 50
Apoptosis, 27, 28, 31, 41, 57, 58
Arthritis, 21, 60
Ascorbic acid, 38, 50
Asthma, 14
Atherosclerosis, 10
Atopic dermatitis, 19, 20, 51, 54, 55
Autoantibodies, 10
Autoimmune diseases, 21, 53
Autoimmunity, 47, 51, 53, 55, 56

B

Barrier function, 47
Basal layer, 47
Benign, 24
Biological therapies, 29
Biomaterials, 62
Biopsy, 36, 37
Blood, 4, 9, 10, 15, 16, 34, 49
Blood circulation, 15
Blood vessels, 4, 15, 34
Bone marrow, 30
Briakinumab, 23, 31, 59

C

Calcipotriol, 24
Calcitriol, 25, 57
Causes, i, iii, v, 7
CD4+, 13, 15, 17, 22, 31, 55, 60
CD8+, 13, 31
CDKAL1, 22, 55, 56
Cell cycle, 41, 58
Cell differentiation, 7, 24, 25, 38
Cellular immunity, 40, 57
Chemokine receptor, 37
Chemokines, 15, 17, 41
Chemotaxis, 29
Chromosome, 18, 19, 20, 21, 53, 54, 55
Classification, 2, 3, 18, 46
Clinical trials, 4, 46
Cluster of differentiation, 9
Coal, 39

Coal tar, 39
Collagen, 37, 62
Combination therapy, 29, 56, 57
Corticosteroids, 23, 24, 25, 26, 56
Cyclosporine, 23, 29, 40, 57, 60
Cytokines, 10, 11, 13, 14, 15, 16, 17, 21, 24, 27, 29, 30, 37, 40, 41, 48, 51, 52, 53

D

Dendritic cell, 4, 13, 14, 15, 22, 40, 52, 63
Dermatitis, 19, 34, 61
Dermatology, 46, 49, 56
Dermatoses, 48, 59
Dermis, 4, 8, 27, 34, 37, 38, 50
Diabetes, 21, 22, 56
Differentiation, 7, 47
DNA, 24, 27, 28, 50
DNA damage, 27, 50

E

Eczema, 61
Efalizumab, 23, 30
Efficacy, 58
Elbows, vii, 3
Elongation, 4
Endothelial cells, 57, 63
Endothelial nitric oxide synthase, 11
Environment, 9
Enzyme, 9, 28, 35, 36, 39, 61
Epidemiology, 45
Epidermis, vii, 4, 5, 7, 11, 16, 18, 19, 26, 27, 37, 38, 39, 46, 47, 48, 50, 60, 61, 63
Erythrocytes, 9, 49
Erythrodermic psoriasis, 3
Etanercept, 23, 30, 46, 51, 58
Etiology, 7, 9, 18
Excimer laser, 57
Extracellular matrix, 38, 63

F

Fibroblasts, 10, 11, 37, 38, 39, 49, 50, 61, 62
Fibronectin, 8
Fungal infection, 30, 31

G

Genes, 17, 18, 19, 20, 22, 24, 25, 29, 37, 51, 54, 55
Genetics, 7, 17, 45, 47, 53, 54
Genome, 17, 20, 53, 54, 55
Glutathione, 9, 52
Growth factor, 9, 16, 58, 60
Guttate psoriasis, 3

H

Heredity, 17
Histology, 4
History, 1, 45, 53
HLA, 9, 13, 16, 18, 35, 53, 60
Homeostasis, 63
Human leukocyte antigen, 9, 13
Hydrocortisone, 24
Hydrogen peroxide, 11, 48
Hydroxyl, 10
Hyperlipidemia, 29
Hyperplasia, 4, 39, 40
Hyperproliferation, 7
Hyperventilation, 26

I

ICAM, 9, 13, 25, 31, 51
IFN, 9, 14, 15, 17, 27, 36, 40, 61
IL-12B, 20
IL-13, 14, 21, 55
IL-17, 14, 17
IL-23R, 20
IL-4, 14, 17, 21, 29
IL-8, 14, 16, 17, 37, 53

Immune response, 18, 22, 41
Immune system, 13, 17, 18, 19, 34, 35, 40
Immunity, 14, 16, 21, 51
Immunoglobulin, 9, 30, 63
Immunopathogenesis, 50, 51, 52
Immunosuppression, 30
In vitro models, 36
Inflammation, 5, 11, 13, 15, 20, 24, 29, 30, 31, 41, 52, 59, 60
Inflammatory bowel disease, 55
Inflammatory cells, 4, 11, 30, 34, 36, 37
Inflammatory disease, 14, 21, 24, 60
Inflammatory mediators, 25, 40
Infliximab, 23, 30, 58, 63, 64
Innate immunity, 14
Integrin, 60, 61
Intercellular adhesion molecule, 9, 13, 25, 51
Involucrin, 8, 36
IP-10, 17

K

Keratin, 9, 25, 47
Keratinocytes, 4, 7, 9, 11, 13, 14, 16, 17, 18, 19, 22, 24, 25, 27, 28, 29, 30, 37, 38, 39, 40, 41, 47, 49, 50, 51, 52, 53, 57, 60, 61, 63
Knees, vii, 3

L

Laminin, 8
Lesions, 3, 11, 15, 16, 27, 30, 40, 50, 51, 56, 61
LFA, 9, 31
Light, 27, 28
Lipid metabolism, 34
Lipid peroxidation, 10, 48, 49
Lipids, 26, 38, 49
Locus, 18, 19, 20, 21, 53, 54
Loricrin, 8
Low-density lipoprotein, 10
Lupus, 21

Lymph node, 15
Lymphocytes, 22, 31
Lymphoid, 11, 15, 21, 51
Lymphoid tissue, 51

M

Macrophages, 33
Major histocompatibility complex, 9, 15
Mast cells, 13, 16, 33, 53
MCP-1, 17
Mechanisms of action, 26, 56
Melanoma, 48
Methotrexate, 23, 28, 57
MHC, 9, 13, 15, 17, 18, 20, 51, 53
Mice, 9, 33, 34, 35, 36, 37, 40, 47, 59, 60, 61, 62
Microcirculation, 63
Microscopy, 48
Migration, 13, 15, 31
Models, vii, 33, 34, 35, 36, 37, 38, 39, 42, 53, 59
Molecules, 14, 15, 26, 28, 40, 58, 63
Monoclonal antibody, 14, 60, 64
Monolayer, 36
mRNA, 11
Mutations, 33, 59

N

Narrowband-UVB, 27
Natural killer cell, 9
Nausea, 26, 28
Neutrophils, 4, 9, 10, 13, 16, 17, 33, 46, 52
Nitric oxide, 9, 10, 11, 49, 50
Nitric oxide synthase, 11, 50

O

Oxidation, 10
Oxidative damage, 9, 10, 50
Oxidative stress, 7, 9, 10, 16, 48, 49

P

Palmoplantar pustulosis, 53
Pathogenesis, 2, 4, 5, 7, 8, 9, 13, 16, 17, 20, 21, 22, 25, 36, 39, 40, 41, 47, 48, 52, 53, 63
Pathology, vii, 1, 4, 33, 42, 61, 63
Pathophysiological, 9
Pathophysiology, 47, 60
Permeability, 4, 26
Peroxidation, 10
Pharmacogenomics, 19
Phenotype, 2, 18, 33, 34, 46, 60, 61
Phototherapy, 23, 26, 27, 28, 62
Placebo, 55
Plaque, 2, 3, 14, 16, 18, 46, 52, 56, 57, 58, 63
Plaque psoriasis, 2
Pneumonia, 28
Polymorphism, 19, 21, 55
Prevalence, 1, 45, 46
Pro-inflammatory, 24, 30, 37
Proliferation, 11, 14, 15, 17, 25, 28, 29, 30, 37, 39, 47, 52, 58, 61, 62, 63
Proteins, 8, 10, 18, 19, 24, 27, 29, 35, 40, 48, 60
Psoralen, 23
Psoriasis, i, iii, v, vii, 1, 2, 3, 4, 7, 9, 10, 11, 12, 13, 14, 16, 17, 18, 19, 20, 21, 22, 23, 24, 25, 26, 27, 28, 29, 30, 33, 34, 35, 36, 37, 39, 40, 41, 42, 45, 46, 47, 48, 49, 50, 51, 52, 53, 54, 55, 56, 57, 58, 59, 60, 61, 62, 63, 64
Psoriatic arthritis, 46, 54, 55, 56, 58
PSORS, 18, 19
Psychological pain, vii, 23
Pustular psoriasis, 3

Q

Quality of life, vii, 4, 23, 42

R

RANTES, 17
Reactive oxygen, 9, 48
Retinoids, 29, 57
Rheumatoid arthritis, 21
Risk, 9, 10, 20, 21, 26, 30, 53, 54, 55
Risk factors, 54
RNA, 50
Rodents, 35

S

Salicylic acid, 23, 26
Self-assembly, 38
Serum, 10, 49, 50
Severity, 3, 46
Side effects, vii, 24, 25, 26, 27, 28, 29, 30, 31, 42
Signal transduction, 9
Signals, 15, 17, 22
Skin, vii, 1, 2, 4, 5, 7, 8, 9, 10, 11, 13, 15, 16, 17, 18, 19, 22, 25, 26, 27, 28, 29, 31, 33, 34, 36, 37, 38, 40, 41, 42, 47, 48, 50, 52, 53, 59, 60, 61, 62, 63
Skin cancer, 27
Skin diseases, 1, 48
SNP, 19
Squamous cell carcinoma, 50
Stress, 10, 48, 49
Substitutes, 38, 62
Susceptibility, 17, 18, 19, 20, 21, 22, 47, 53, 54, 55, 56
Symptoms, vii, 16, 23, 26, 30, 31, 42

T

T cell intracellular signaling, 21
T cells, 13-17, 20, 21, 22, 24, 25, 28, 29, 31, 33, 34, 37, 38, 40, 41, 51, 52, 56, 59, 60
T cells activity, 13
T helper cells (Th), 13
T lymphocytes, 4, 40, 46, 52
Tar, 26, 57

Tazarotene, 23, 25
TGF, 35, 60
Th cells, 14
Th1/Th2/Th17 balance, 14, 15
Th17 pathway, 13, 14, 17, 20
Therapy, 24, 26-28, 34, 39, 40, 46, 56, 57, 58
Three-dimensional model, 38
Thymus, 21, 34
Tissue, 9, 11, 15, 16, 41, 61, 62
TNF, 9-11, 13, 14, 17, 27, 30, 37, 40, 50, 60
Topical treatments, 24, 56
Toxicity, 26, 28, 29, 40
Transglutaminase, 8
Transplant, 34
Treatment, 3, 4, 14, 19, 20, 24-30, 39, 40, 41, 45, 46, 52, 56, 57, 58, 63, 64

U

Ustekinumab, 20, 23, 31
UV irradiation, 26

V

Vascularization, 33, 35, 36
Vessels, 5
Vitamin A, 25, 29, 50
Vitamin D, 24, 26, 56
Vitamin D analogues, 23, 25
Vitamin E, 9

W

Wavelengths, 27
Wound healing, 63

X

Xenotransplantation, 34

Z

ZNF313, 21, 22, 55